EWALD'S WISDOM

For reviews contact the author at simonbsr@gmail.com

First edition published in 2025 by
Blockhouse Books
ISBN 978-10370-3262-22
Cover design, graphics and page layout by Wim Rheeder
Set in 11 point on 16 point, Barlow
Printed and bound by Castle Graphics, Cape Town

Cover Image: Langvlei, near Sedgefield, Western Cape, looking towards George Peak.

EWALD'S WISDOM

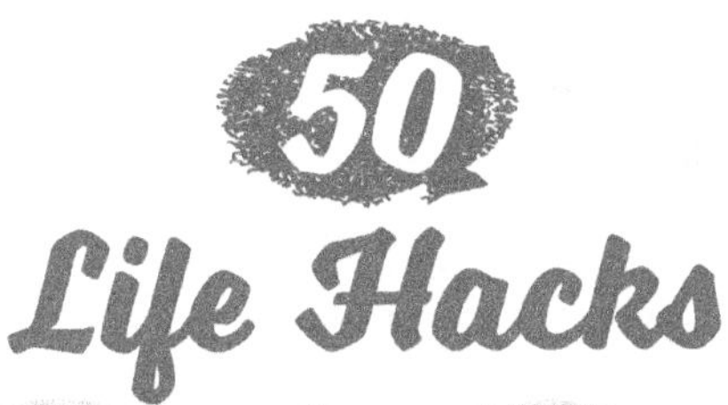

FOR MIND, BODY & SOUL

SIMON C GREEN

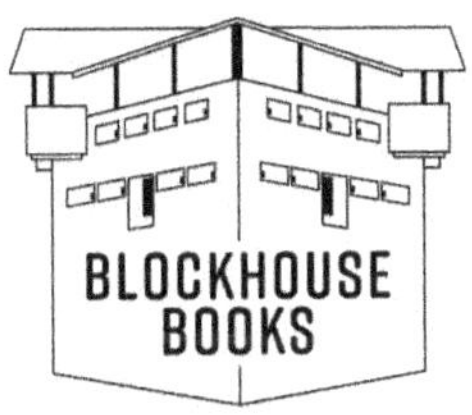

Endorsements

"This book is more than a guide - it is an invitation. An invitation to step into a life of conscious awareness, to embrace the wisdom of those who have walked before us, and to recognise the power within ourselves to heal, transform, and transcend. And perhaps, just perhaps, those who seek a life-changing shift, a new way of being, will find inspiration within these pages. Some may even feel called to take their rightful place within the Body Stress Release family, contributing to an ever-growing collective of wisdom keepers. May you read these pages not just with your mind, but with your heart open to the possibility of change. And may you walk away from this book not only informed but forever inspired."

Dr. Melody Fourie

Holistic Health Practitioner & Friend of BSR

"As someone who has dedicated my life to growth - both in business and personal transformation - I truly believe that wisdom is one of the most powerful tools we have. That's why Ewald's Wisdom: 50 Life Hacks for Mind, Body and Soul resonated so deeply with me. This book embodies that same principle - helping us realign, release what no longer serves us, and step into our fullest potential."

Anthea Vorster

Growth By Design, Business Change Catalyst, & Friend of BSR

"More than just a book, Ewald's Wisdom is a compass - a practical guide to navigating life with clarity, awareness, and purpose. Whether through adjusting one's mindset, refining physical health, or deepening spiritual insight, the wisdom within these pages offers a timeless gift to all who seek it. Simon's own experiences weave through the narrative, adding depth, authenticity, and relatability - ensuring that each lesson is not just read, but felt."

Thomas W E Budge
Clinical Hypnotherapist, Author, & Lifestyle Coach

"More often than not I would be left scratching my head after an 'interesting' chat with Ewald and it has been fascinating to get Simon's perspective on these pearls of wisdom. Credit to Simon for embracing one of Ewald's' wisdoms, and that is one of 'allowingness'. Simon has created the space within his book for those of all backgrounds, religions and world views to enjoy these incredibly practical life hacks. Ewald undeniably had the gift of viewing life from a loftier perspective, and I for one am grateful that these wisdoms can be shared far and wide."

Sandy Damant
BSR Practitioner and Academy Instructor

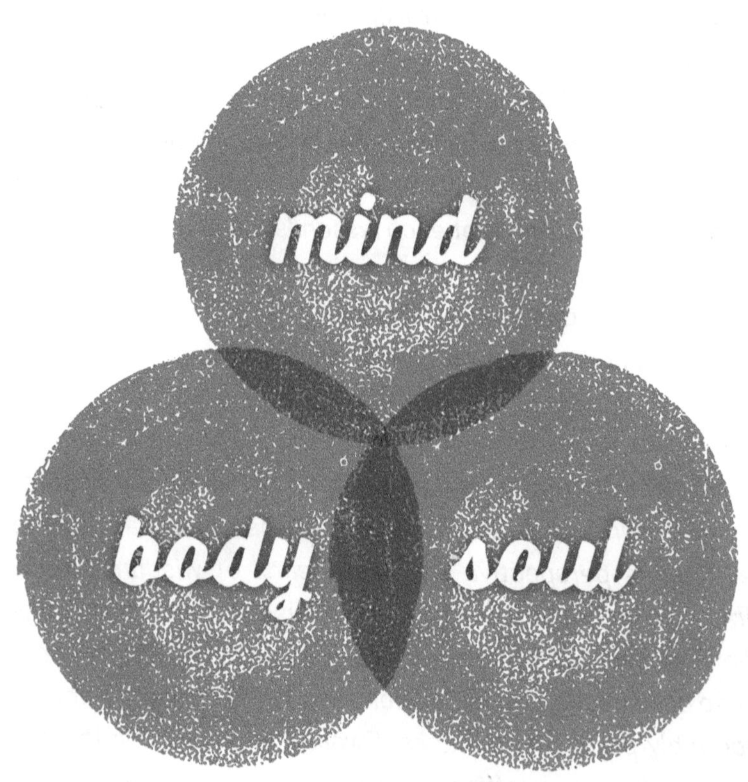
mind
body
soul

Contents

Foreword 9
Preface 11
Introduction 17
Ewald Meggersee - His Life Story 19
What is Body Stress Release? 26

The Mind

#1. Innovation is key 33
#2. Develop a sense of refreshment and energy 37
#3. Beware of boredom 41
#4. Adopt a state of oneness 45
#5. My full potential self is the real me! 49
#6. Thinking is dangerous. Knowing, is joy and pleasure 53
#7. Keep it simple! 57
#8. Have an enquiring mind 61
#9. We do not see the world as it is, but as we are 65
#10. The World as abundance 69
#11. Don't fix what is wrong, work on what's right 73
#12. Make the effort to become effortless 77
#13. Emotions bring the largest discord to humanity 81
#14. Where the mind is focused, energy flows 85
#15. Be Open 89
#16. Ego alert! 93
#17. 'Allowingness' 97
#18. Never judge others 101
#19. Let Intuition 'sneak in' 105

The Body

#20. See the body as whole and complete 113
#21. Stress creates deficiencies 117
#22. Mask on first 121
#23. The need for rest 125

#24. The body doesn't know how to lie 129
#25. Listen to your body 133
#26. The body makes the best of a bad situation 137
#27. Exercise with wisdom, think with clarity 141
#28. Body's wisdom is more powerful than the mind 145
#29. The body is natural "detoxer" 149
#30. Daily re-energising 153
#31. Love from the heart 157
#32. The body loves gentleness 161
#33. Everything in its time 165
#34. Moderation is everything 169
#35. The body has the strictest discipline 173
#36. Resonate with yourself 177
#37. The heart knows 181
#38. Honour your body 185

The Soul

#39. Develop a sense of joy 193
#40. Your beliefs determine your reality 197
#41. No self-judgement 201
#42. You receive what you give 205
#43. Pay attention to your dreams 209
#44. Intention needs to be pure 213
#45. Your beliefs limit your achievements 217
#46. Never lose sight of the bigger picture 221
#47. Healing comes from above-down, and inside-out 225
#48. Earn the right to tap into higher frequencies 229
#49. Stand in your own power 233
#50. Everything with Spiritual Wisdom 237

Acknowledgements 240
Final Word from Ewald 242
Bibliography 243
Other media 246
Websites 247
A selection of Ewald's Preferred Reading 249
Titles also available by Simon C Green 250

Foreword

50 Life Hacks for Mind, Body, and Soul based on Ewald's Wisdom - what a lovely project Simon has taken on. Wisdom is a quality of the soul, where the heart qualities of kindness, care, compassion, empathy, and love are important. If those qualities can be brought to bear on our daily physical, mental, and emotional struggles and challenges, that would be wisdom in practice; those would be great life hacks.

I met Ewald in 1986 after a severe whiplash in a motor accident and became a regular client, and after a few years, a close friend of Ewald and Gail Meggersee. My wife Jane and I found we shared a common interest with them in the deeper things in life, we meditated together regularly and shared our inner experiences and, in the early days of our friendship, travelled together to meet mystics and 'wise ones' that came across our path. These included meeting Michael Roads at the Omega Institute in New York, a disciple of the 'Magus of Strovolos' in Cyprus, and Mother Meera in Germany.

In Ewald's spiritual journey, he was influenced early on by the clairvoyant Edgar Cayce and he was also interested in other-dimensional existences and supernormal phenomena such as UFOs and aliens. He often spoke about them to the bemusement of more earth-bound people, like me.

As co-founder, with Gail of the profession of Body Stress Release, Ewald would teach the philosophy module of the practitioner training course. This gave him the opportunity to shake the conditioned thinking of students often emphasising the oneness of all existence and the illusionary nature of separation that most of us are trapped in.

At times, Ewald experienced expanded awareness. He often had a wider perspective of situations thanks to this ability. One of his oft-repeated comments was, *"Always look at the bigger picture!"* With our conditioned minds our view is often limited by our life experience and he saw things from a higher vantage point. That, I think, was the source of his wisdom, which shone through in his many sayings. And those sayings are what Simon has latched onto and developed in this book, adding his own wisdom drawn from his life experiences.

Wisdom has come to humanity from many sources over the ages. I think we all have a "wisdom detector" somewhere in our heart or our gut. We know it when we meet it. It rings true. I am sure that your wisdom detector will be buzzing as you read Simon's interpretation of Ewald's Wisdom. May your life be uplifted (hacked?) by it!

Boetie Toerien
BSR Practitioner and Academy Instructor

Preface

Finding myself in The Wilderness

I never imagined that having a career-changing event would mean going to the wilderness, but actually, it did. Not THE wilderness, but Wilderness, a small town in the Western Cape of South Africa. In 2015, I went to the Academy of Body Stress Release to train for five months to become a qualified Body Stress Release (BSR) Practitioner. I then established my own practice in Johannesburg and for the first time ever worked for myself! It really was a liberating moment, but it took me 37 years to get there. As I tell everyone, if you are happy with where you are today - then you have to know that both the good AND the bad were essential in bringing you to that happiness by shaping your life. So, perhaps understanding how I got to this point in writing a book about someone I never met, might just help you understand me a little better.

I have many friends who started their own business, either as a consultant or forming their own companies, and thought *"That sounds great, wonderful, challenging, scary... Yikes! That's not for me!"* I had been 'Mr Salary Man' working for three large corporates ever since leaving the British Army in 2006. This journey to becoming a BSR Practitioner was the next career pivot on my journey through life.

Army Life prepared me for continuous change

I am a late Baby Boomer, born in 1958, so thirty years in the Army should have molded me into sticking to one specialisation, one sector, one BIG idea for my work. Well, no actually, it did not, actually quite the opposite. The one thing I did learn in the Army is that nothing ever stays the same on this journey we call life, and change is the oxygen I need to flourish. Military service prepared me very well to cope with life 'on the outside', for any challenge, big or small. On leaving the Army, after a life of high-impact technology, I became a consultant working back into areas of the military I was familiar with, working with loyal ex-army colleagues. My first career pivot was to take the systems engineering expertise I had had in communications technology and apply that to Army uniforms! Yes, you really can do that, it was ground-breaking work, taking combat uniform, usually procured as individual items, which quite often failed to fit together and applying a systems engineering approach - with a 'human-in-the-loop' for the ergonomic aspect. I loved it - all 'New Stuff'. It was an easy transition, and one I really appreciated, and life in London at that point was pretty idyllic. But a previous military assignment in South Africa was to bring me back to the southern hemisphere quite quickly.

Aircraft Development

I received a phone call one day of a job offer, which 48 hours later, took me to an interview in Copenhagen Airport, and within 6 weeks I was packing my bags to emigrate lock, stock, and barrel to South Africa. I was offered a Key Account Manager's job in the aerospace manufacturing sector, working for Denel Aerostructures, career pivot number two. I spent a challenging and wonderful time there during an exciting aircraft development phase for the A400M military airlifter. I managed three work packages as the Programme Director. However, after four hectic and very creative years in high-tech manufacturing, the need for a change took me in a different direction once again and into another new sector. The Chief Aircraft Designer, Eli asked me *"What do you know about the Security Sector, Simon? You're successful here, why leave now, don't you think you should stay?"* For the very reason I made a success of one new sector, was why I was doing it all over again, this time at a Profit and Loss level, in the private sector. Career pivot number three.

Cut and thrust of the Security Business in Africa

The position in G4S as the General Manager for their Technology Business Unit took my career as a corporate executive to the next level, both in terms of profit and loss delivery and, of course, stress too. This was also getting noticed at home; long hours and managing two company retrenchment schemes to "streamline the business" was taking its toll. A year after the disastrous London Olympic Games contract losses for G4S and some other economic challenges for the FTSE 100 listed Company, savings had to be made and I was retrenched at 55. No pivot this time unless it was to be the scrap heap!

Retrenchment and Reflection

The dreaded retrenchment is something I would never recommend to anyone! I was a white, middle-aged foreigner, at executive level and five years away from official retirement age in a country striving for employment equity - post apartheid. Not a great position to find myself in, and it could have been my second midlife crisis. For the next 18 months, I took an ambivalent approach to finding a job, licking my wounds and ignoring my mantra that 'finding a job, is a full-time job.' I improved my LinkedIn profile, became a Premium Member, and waited for the offers to flood in. I did get offers, don't get me wrong, but the Middle East and a few other hot spots around the World were not what I really had in mind. I had come to South Africa to live and work here, with a new family, not to then work somewhere else. Even in the global workplace, home is where the heart is, and that was in edgy Johannesburg.

I took time to finish off a writing project, did some creative courses in photography and writing, and became more spiritual in my relationship with God. Financial security at home and a very understanding and well-salaried wife led me into a wonderful period of self-discovery. I got to know my 8-year-old boy so much better! Unfortunately though, hours at the computer writing and researching gave me very bad backache, together with neck and shoulder pains.

Years in the armed forces had provided my body, like so many others in the office and corporate environment, with a good physical coping mechanism. Some exercise, a bit of sport, the odd stretch and visits to the podiatrists, chiropractor, doctors, and Pilates classes had all managed to suppress the pains over the years. In addition to my wife being financially supportive of the situation, she is also the nagging guardian of my health, in a nice way of course! She needs me healthy - we run, hike, and cycle every challenge in life together and it makes us stronger, at least up to the point I start to struggle.

A Life-Changing Moment

"Get fixed right now" was the clear message, from my wife, and the offer I could not refuse was a visit to a Body Stress Release Practitioner. Together we tripped off to visit Brent Garvie in Johannesburg to have our first BSR session. We sat down in his practice, and I was immediately told to sit up straight and not to cross my legs - oh no! I was back in school, this time posture school. After taking my physical life history in a few minutes,

Brent got to work.

Body Stress Release works on the principle that any form of mechanical, mental or chemical stress is stored where the stress manifests, and thus can be released using various precise points on the body. The session only takes 30 minutes and is completed fully clothed. Brent told me, *"Now you need to go home, rest, get horizontal and don't do anything physical till I see you again in three days' time."*

By the time I had driven home I felt like I had completed the 109km Cape Argus Cycle Race, which usually takes me about 5 hours. I went into a deep sleep that afternoon. There was something to this Body Stress Release. Over the next few weeks, all my aches and pains vanished. Little did I realise that I was actually healing myself. Deep and nagging leg pains from my hips to my feet had gone and I returned to full fitness in about 6 weeks. I also learned Brent's life story, and his journey to becoming a practitioner. I did more research and looked into the practitioner course availability. After all, I was at a crossroads, and definitely not yet retired and on the scrap heap, but still not working and earning a living. Brent had already asked me *"Why don't you become a BSR Practitioner?"* The little 'Doubting Thomas' from within was still whispering, *"What do you know about health and wellness, and working for yourself is hard you know?"* Well, I had changed sectors three times before, so why not again? Another few weeks later, and my business plan was ready, I had written my web pages, sourced a practice location and I started the course on May Day, 2015. Career pivot number four, into health and wellness. Last one right?

I don't think my body and stress story is unique, I think it fully typifies the world we live in; poor diets, low levels of physical activity and stressful high-paced lifestyles, which mean we all get stressed out, and one day you might be my client in Johannesburg!

The Body Stress Release Course is amazing, comprising 5 months of taught study and practical training with about twenty other students from all over the world. It is held in an idyllic spot on the Garden Route, but in the winter! Whoa! It got cold in my mountain lodge in the valley there, but the course was fun and a powerful way to start my next life pivot. The course teachers were brilliant, and at that time the course was taught by one of the BSR Founders, Gail Meggersee, but her husband, Ewald, who had also taught the course up until 2011, had already passed away. Gail and Ewald had been an amazing team and it was clear from my course and subsequent years in practice, that they were very different individuals and had had very different impacts on BSR and in teaching their students. I would often hear *"Oh that was Ewald's saying"* or *"Ewald really believed in that"*,... but who was Ewald? And what was his story? We're about to find out in the next section.

Did I say I was done pivoting? Well my last one to date, number 5, has been to become a non-fiction writer and self-published author. I have written two books on the Anglo-Boer War Blockhouses, in South Africa and, and of course, this book. History, heritage, and telling stories has become my passion; I even put my own BSR practice on the back-burner, though I had been fully committed to being the Chairperson of the South African Association of BSR up until 2025. Next career pivot...? Irons are certainly in the fire... my story is to be continued.

Introduction

I hope you know me a little by now, but do you know the real me? What makes me tick, and in asking that about myself - what of you? Ask yourself - Who am I? It's not about where you were born, if you are married or single or what your job is etc. No, it's deeper than that. After being retrenched here is what I came up with to describe who I am.

I **trust in God** for all my being, He is in control - for you though, it can be another version of the 'higher universal power' out there.

Have fun daily in all I do. If it stops being fun, I stop doing it.

I **learn daily**, through all media in order to keep moving progressively forward in a state of constant change.

I seek to influence and **inspire others**, through my connectivity to other people, in any way possible to help them in their own journey. I live my life through others.

I seek continuously to use my time, talents, and treasures to **give to others**, without expectations.

This book takes 50 of Ewald's great one-liners, some might not be his exclusively, but often his mantra nevertheless, and the ones he applied to his life and to teaching Body Stress Release. They have been sorted into our three key elements; mind, body, and soul. The writing is also, quite naturally, a part of me too, and my interpretation from my 60-plus years of life and its own ups and downs. In that regard, I will never do Ewald total justice as a second-hand recorder who didn't know the man. However, that said, I'll do my best to capture something, and rest assured his wisdom has been passed to me through the teaching of the BSR technique. In the words of his great friend and colleague Boetie Toerien, *"He was more in the moment, in the heart, than in the head."* Let's enjoy his wisdom, with my own take on it, and my experience as a BSR practitioner added for good measure, and see where it takes us on our journey together.

In using the book, feel free to read from page 1 to page 250 or dip in using the contents page for a topic that pricks your attention or flick through and see what captures your eye; a random page selection might also work. My basic desire is to change the world for the better. In that haughty mission, and from you reading this book, I have only to inspire or help one person on their journey to achieve my purpose. Making a difference is that simple. Using the principle that we apply in Body Stress Release, that the body takes what it needs from the technique and disregards the rest, please do the same in reading this book, take what you need and simply ignore the rest. I hope you take more than you disregard.

I am undeniably and unapologetically a Christian, I know from first-hand accounts Ewald did believe in a higher power, and a God, though did not necessarily attend church or read the Bible. In his Principles Class of 2010 he taught *"I am divine principle and law; I am divine abundance; and I am perfect."* The word 'divine' being defined as "connected with a god, or like a god" (Cambridge Dictionary Online). If the biblical quotes are not for you please skip over them, I respect that completely. Or treat them just as nice words from a good storybook. You will notice in the wisdom quotes I have taken them from the widest sources possible. I hope you enjoy the book and please feel free to give me feedback, on the email address on the imprint page. Now you need to understand who Ewald was, before we get to the wisdom of his words.

Ewald Meggersee -
His Life Story

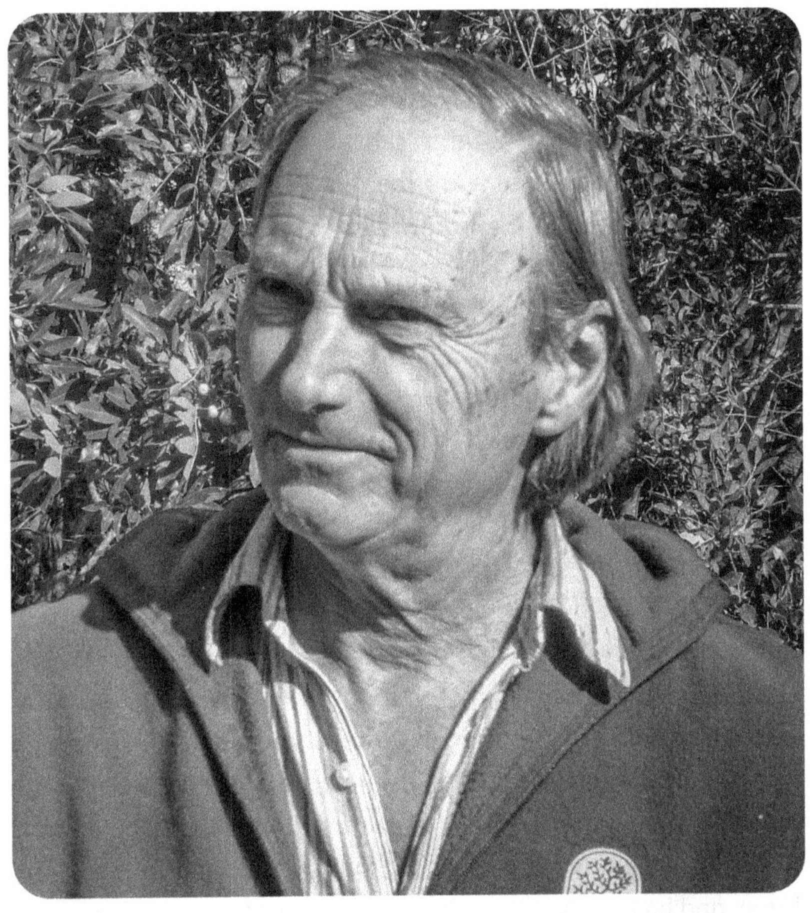

Ewald Meggersee (1944-2013)
(Photo courtesy of Jeanette Gibbs)

Of course, for those who do not practice BSR, or have never even heard of the technique, you will not know of Ewald Meggersee, and will ask "Who is Ewald?" Well, here is his life story in brief to set the scene for his wisdom to come.

He was born the Eastern Cape (former Transkei) in 1944 to parents who owned a trading store, where he grew up as a free-spirited child, speaking Xhosa and playing in the red African soil. Before technology, boys used to climb trees, and one day aged 5, the adventurous Ewald fell from one, rendering him unconscious. When he woke-up a week later, sadly his life had changed for the worse, and he started to suffer continuous shooting pains in his legs, deep burning in the lower back, numb hands and a raft of other body complications. Back in the post-World War Two era, sympathy was a rare commodity, as everyone was digging deep to recover and trying to get their lives back to normal. Ewald was told it was *"All in his imagination,"* and no doubt to *"Stop complaining."* As a parent myself, I've said that many times of course.

In later years, however, his school life became a nightmare, due to the constant pain he felt. He could not sit still and the burning sensations in the feet led him to take off his shoes and socks regularly. He was quickly labelled an 'attention seeker', and one of the 'naughty boys'. Boys in the South African psyche all had to be sporty! But this was also nightmare for the now-teenage Ewald, where constant stiffness and pain prevented him from doing very much at all. Forced into sports, he underperformed which led to a feeling of humiliation and lack of self-confidence. Other elements of his schooling were also impacted, such as life in the cadet force, and he claimed to be the first boy ever to be 'dishonourably discharged'. The pains and issues were just not going way.

Sadly, the medical profession wasn't managing to diagnose the correct cause and treatment for his condition either. The symptoms were obvious and acute, as many BSR practitioners have witnessed in their own practice clients, but the root cause was impossible to discern at this stage. X-Rays showed nothing wrong, misdiagnosis of his aching back as kidney pain and the consequent penicillin medication failed to help the ailing Ewald. At one point he was also referred to a psychologist, believing it was still 'all in his head'. As you might expect, all of this had a traumatic effect on the young and emerging adult.

The constant pain led him to withdraw from his peers, and he became a quiet and introspective young man, searching for the answers from within himself. Withdrawn into an emotional corner, little did he know at the time that his own body really held the answer to, and relief from, his locked-in body stress. Ewald's purpose in the world would soon start to develop and blossom, and two things led to this - the freedom of university life and meeting his future wife, Gail.

By now Ewald, the young adult, was better at masking his pain, and he threw himself into university life, playing rugby, building sets for the university theatre, and even started to weight train to strengthen his back. His search for the answers within also led him to be 'Ewald the Philosopher', which meant he always 'questioned the conventional'. Up to this point the conventional was not providing answers and treatments for the continuous aches and pains, so this questioning was only natural for him.

Gail and Ewald's relationship blossomed and they were married, both graduating from university and heading off to Cape Town to start married life. Ewald worked as an industrial chemist and Gail a French teacher. Sadly though, his symptoms became even more severe, often waking at night with screams of pain and jumping out of bed hopping around the floor clutching his cramped calf as if it were snapped in two. The theatre-loving Gail would ask him unsympathetically; *"Do you have to be so dramatic?"* His health continued to decline with a range of allergies and now his body frequently collapsed on him. He feared being paralysed and wheelchair bound for the rest of his life. Medical interventions continued to fail and the proposals for exploratory surgery were declined by him as being too risky and radical.

Then came some hope! The relatively new medical technique of chiropractic, developed in America at the turn of the 19th century was recommended to Ewald, and he started to get some relief at long last. Albeit the relief only lasted a few days and his back was strangely tighter, he felt it was a start to his healing process. Little did he know his healing process was one the world needed to learn about and appreciate too. The difference though was so marked, and the couple so impressed, that they considered becoming chiropractors themselves. There were, however, many obstacles preventing them, not least of which was moving all the way to America in the 1970s, as the education of chiropractors was banned in South Africa. Ultimately, it was Gail who asked the question *"Why not?"* that spurred them on to head off on their adventure and ultimately change the world for very many people.

In 1977, they landed in South Carolina and became penniless students again to study chiropractic medicine at Sherman College of Straight Chiropractic. They had enough cash to pay for their initial tuition fees and rent a meagre place to stay off-the-beaten track. For other 'luxuries' such as furniture, Ewald made these from reclaimed wood he sourced from scrap heaps. Gail the resourceful woman she was, scavenged the rest and they made a comfortable home to withstand the harsh heat and bitter winters of South Carolina.

Life was hard for the Meggersees, they worked two jobs, studied and made the best of a new life in America. Unfortunately, the chiropractic technique experienced at the college was far too harsh for Ewald's sensitive back and often he would end up almost paralysed due to its application, the pain in many instances escalating. Gail attended many of the visiting lecturer's seminars in a search for a 'something else' remedy and maybe something a little less harsh. It was on one of these seminars that she had the good fortune to meet Doctor Richard van Rumpt. He was a qualified chiropractor but one who adopted a very different approach to the more traditional approach. His Directional None-Force Technique's (DNFT) title resonated with the astute Gail, declaring to Ewald after attending his class; *"Here lies the truth"*, and the clue was in the title. The Van Rumpt technique was what BSR was to become, a gentle, precise "non-force" modality. It was this meeting that was to prove the catalyst for the establishment of the Body Stress Release technique as global brand several years later. The Meggersees returned to South Africa in 1981 as qualified chiropractors and armed with Van Rumpt's DNFT teachings.

They opened a practice in Claremont, Cape Town and very quickly established themselves a thriving practice, established by success and word-of-mouth referrals. They applied their knowledge in a unique way and soon out of several years of heuristic development, (which might be commonly referred to as 'trial and error') incredible results were achieved. Along the way no greater application was made than on Ewald himself, whom Gail called *"the ultimate guinea pig"* and eventually the ultimate success story in his own personal healing journey. He gradually became more flexible and one day woke in a state of dread - something was missing! For the first time in his memorable life, Ewald was pain-free, and Ewald got his life back. Years later in 2019, in my own practice I had a client tell me the same thing after two sessions of BSR she said *"I've had a headache for over 30 years and now it's gone - what did you do?"*

Their success however hadn't gone unnoticed and the two factions of chiropractic; the 'mixer' and the 'straight' factions were under pressure from the government in South Africa to *"...speak with one voice."* Previously the Department of Health had closed the Chiropractic Register, and was not, in the mid-1980s, prepared to reopen it. Technically the Meggersees and about 40 others who had trained overseas were practising illegally. Although this was a technicality, it was soon clear that the Meggersees were being singled out as scapegoats, and were charged with operating illegally and summoned to appear at the local police station, their practice now closed. When they left the Police station, however, Ewald calmly took his next client, and continued to practice.

Their court case was delayed several times through a successful letter-writing campaign by their loyal clients, but in the end they were refused their chiropractic registration, but not prosecuted. The proviso in the judgement was that they start their own modality and stop being part of traditional medicine. By now, the fledgling technique of Body Stress Release was ready to be born to the world. They relaunched their practice as Body Stress Release and in 1987 taught their first BSR course in Claremont, Cape Town, to six former clients. Over the ensuing years fifty-five practitioners of BSR were trained at their Claremont practice until 1996 when they moved to the country on South Africa's Garden Route, to a small place called Rondevlei, aptly near a town called Wilderness. Subsequent training courses were held in Rondevlei, and are still run there today.

They formed the Body Stress Release Association of South Africa and up until Ewald's retirement in 2011 they had together taught over 334 BSR practitioners who practise worldwide. Today, the modality is a flourishing global organisation spanning over 20 countries, with four governing associations and around 700 BSR practitioners having been trained.

Sadly, the Meggersees separated and a few years later in 2013, Ewald died, followed by Gail in 2021. Their ashes were scattered on the property they owned together in Rondevlei, which had become the Body Stress Release Academy of South Africa. No doubt their souls look down on every new student taught there on the annual course for new practitioners.

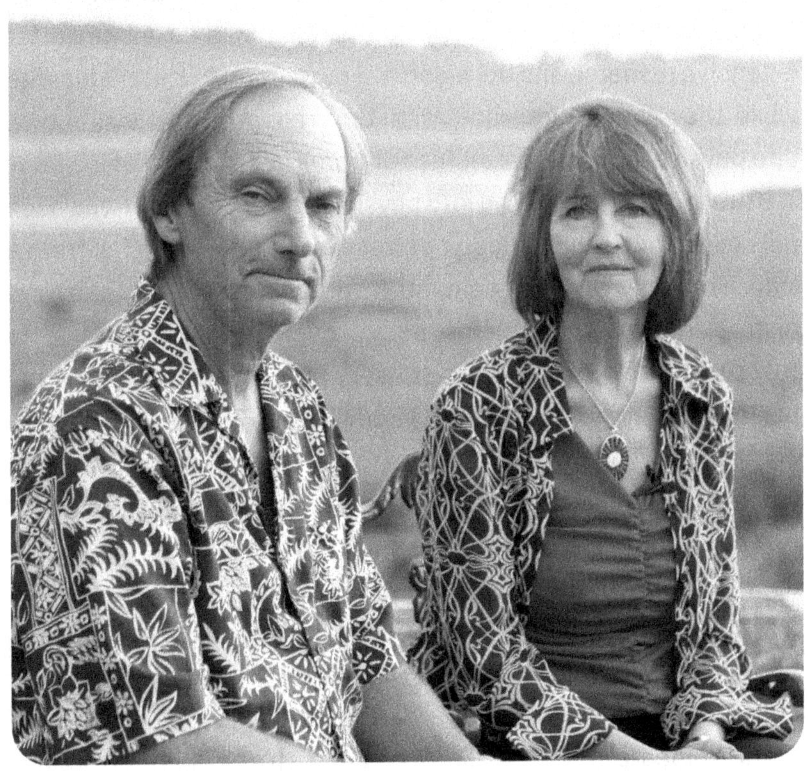

Ewald and Gail Meggersee at the BSR Academy, Rondevlei, WC.
(Photo courtesy of Marie Stone)

What is Body Stress Release?

Body Stress Release is a non-therapeutic complementary health-care modality. It is concerned with assisting the body to release stored tension, thereby allowing it to maximise its in-built ability to maintain and heal itself. This technique has been developed and practised in South Africa since 1981 and was developed after extensive research and development by Gail and Ewald Meggersee while they were chiropractors, and in response to Ewald's own dire physical adversity after his fall from a tree as a child.

Stress becomes locked into physical structures when the body fails to adapt to an overload of stress, such as Ewald's fall from a tree. This may result in pain, stiffness, numbness, and postural distortions. In addition, the body's capacity to undertake its functions, such as digestion, sensory processing, and hormonal balancing may be undermined. Body Stress Release is a gentle procedure which works in areas of the body where stress is located, using the body as a biofeedback mechanism to test for it. The practitioner assists the body to release the tension by applying light but definite pressure to the sites of body stress.

The BSR technique is a purely physical modality, designed to help the body release its stored tensions. With the person fully clothed and lying down, the practitioner carries out a series of tests to locate the exact sites of body stress, and determines the precise directions in which the lines of tension exist. This is done by applying light pressure to various points on the body, and observing muscular responses. In this way, the body acts as a biofeedback mechanism, supplying the information required. By working on the physical body, there is however, an accepted understanding that there is also an interaction and impact on the mind and soul components.

The practitioner then applies a light but definite pressure, in the exact directions necessary to encourage the body to release the stored tension.

When the locked-in stress is released, there is a return of the normal life energy flow, this may occur immediately or gradually, in stages, depending on how long the tension has been present in the body. As this is a process, a minimum of 3 appointments will initially be setup. The first session typically lasts approximately one hour, while follow-up sessions are between 30 to 45 minutes.

If you would like to find a practitioner anywhere in the world, there is a Find a Practitioner button on its main website at: www.bodystressrelease.com/

Body Stress Release

Unlocking tension
Restoring self-healing

BSR is a non-therapeutic, complementary approach to health. It does not involve the diagnosis or treatment of any illness, condition or defect and is not a substitute for any treatment of any kind, medical or otherwise.

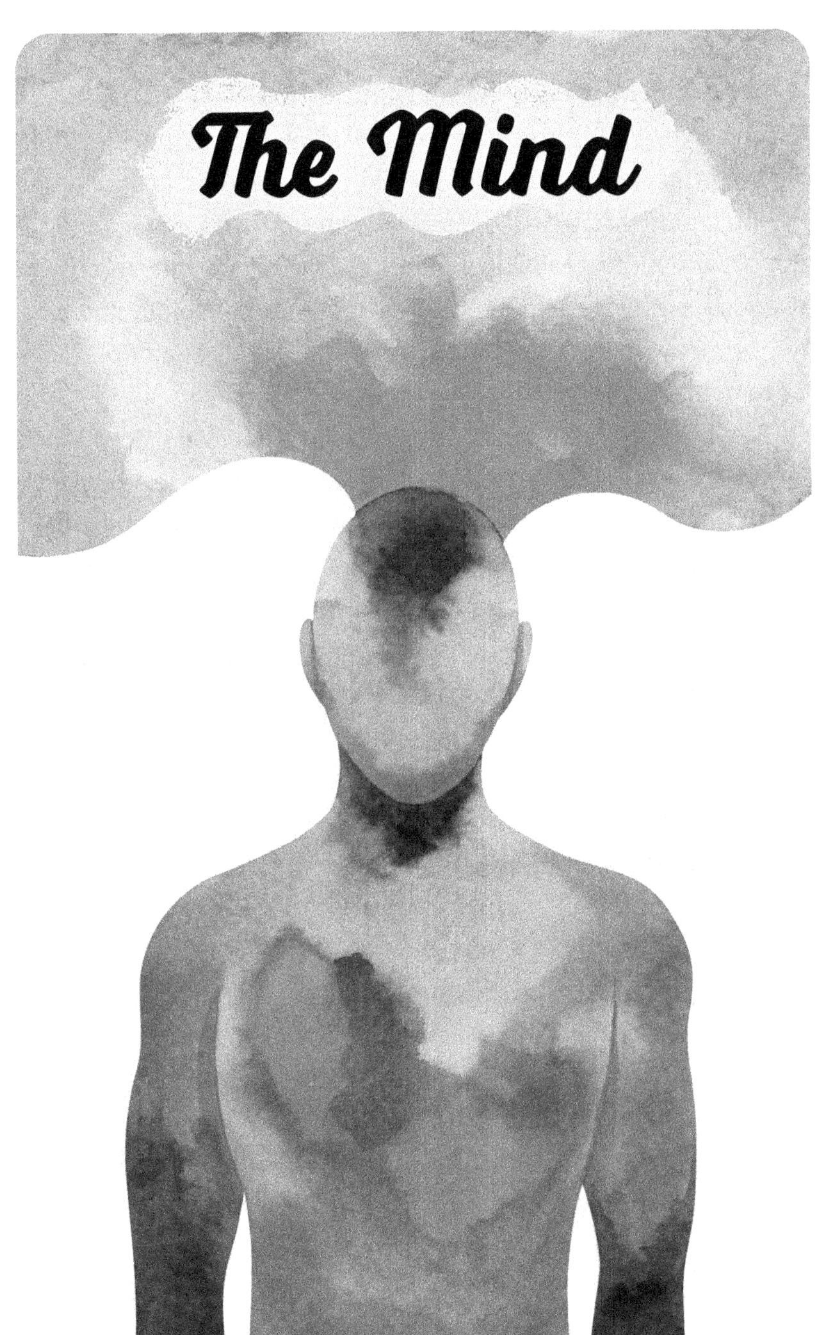
The Mind

We like to imagine that our brains are this homogenous entity that knows and controls everything we do. It processes data, stores information, builds experience, and allows us to navigate our lives. In the background it runs all bodily systems programmed by some higher entity into our DNA. Our body does all manner of things without us realising most of the time, with the majority of the brain's activity being in the realm of sub-conscious thought. Consciously we know very little of what our body and our brain is up to. A bit scary really.

But physically our body also stores processing power and intelligence in other parts of the body. Let's take the reflex action, put your hand on something hot and when the hand jumps off - the action is initiated by brain cells or 'grey-matter' in the spine. It's an involuntary response, the brain would react too slowly, and our hand would be badly burnt if it were allowed to process the pain sensation first and then react to it. This aspect has played an important part in ensuring humanity's survival, as it allows quick reaction to certain dangerous threats. This part of the brain, termed the Reptilian Brain (or Basal Ganglia) handles these survival instincts and autonomic behaviours.

Conceptually, but not physically, we have two other brains in the body; the heart where our emotions are processed, and the gut which deals with instincts and intuition. Let's go to our love place - the heart, or the Paleomammalian Brain (or Limbic System) which manages emotions and also controls the memory and smell. Symbolised by the heart emoji, it really is the place of love, but also the place where ALL emotions reside, the lovely fluffy-cloud ones, we love to feel and also the not so easy to deal with emotions such as hate, greed, jealousy, anxiety, ego, and sadness. They come in 'Yin and Yang' pairs and for every positive one there is a negative. Some of these we are in control of, but others we are not, for example; it can be really tricky to hide when you are really emotionally surprised. Our faces give it away to those observing us.

The opportunity to exploit our inner emotional selves was first brought to light in the 1960s and sprung onto the world by Daniel Goleman, and his bestselling book, *Emotional Intelligence*. In addition to having a measurable level intelligence as an IQ or Intelligence Quotient, we can now be measured in terms of our EQ or Emotional Quotient. Defined as *"the ability to understand, use, and manage your own emotions in positive ways to relieve stress, communicate effectively, empathise with others, overcome challenges, and defuse conflict."* Pretty useful in many situations and all are heart and emotionally centred.

Go on say it *"I knew intuition would be last!"* - well that's intuition, the ability to understand and act on something instinctively, without the need for conscious reasoning. It can be more than an understanding, it can be a physical feeling. Just like the 'broken-heart' feeling in our chests, you can get a feeling deep in the gut. You've literally had that 'gut feeling' about something, and we'll deal with more of this concept in the later 'wisdoms'.

Let's do a worked example to show just how these three "brains" work in a given situation, as they are all in competition.

You meet someone at a party, and they are attractive, well-dressed and personable; the emotional heart is piqued; *"umm cute, we're interested."* It whispers inside you. As the talk progresses this person is really rude to the waiter in a quite demeaning way.

Gut-intuition says, *"Hey heart, hang on, something's wrong here!"* Houston, we have a problem! There is a conflict going on, but watch out, here comes the logical brain to sort it all out for you.

The brain says, *"Well maybe this person is having a bad day.*

Surely, heart it was once off? this person can't be so rude all the time , can they?" The rational brain is busy sorting this conflict out when the attractive person, gazing into your non-attentive eyes says *"Hey would you like to come out to dinner"*... What is your answer? - which brain wins?

Heart is saying *"Oh yeah! Let's go"*; guts says *"No way José"*; and the brain says *"Maybe you'll be fine, you should go right?"* And these three brain intelligences compete and do this to us ALL the time...

#1

Innovation is key

"I am always ready to learn, although I do not always like being taught."

Winston Churchill (1874-1965)
British statesman, military officer, and writer who was Prime Minister of the United Kingdom from 1940 to 1945 and 1951 to 1955.

"...just because something has never been done before does not mean it cannot be done..."

Christie Golden (1963-present) from Rise of the Horde
American fantasy, horror, and sci-fi author.

"We have forgotten how to see anew, the way a child sees, everything brimming with the excitement of discovery. We have labelled and categorized everything, and we have lost the newness of seeing."

Michael J Roads (1937-2024)
UK-born resident of Australia, best-selling author.

It was Ewald's view that you should *"be open to learning, from every aspect of life..."* So why do we learn? Usually, it is to acquire new knowledge or skills, starting at school and then maybe through further education. But it doesn't stop there as many graduates believe. Now, we are in an era of 'life-long learning', which is a continuous process. Even the task of keeping pace with the latest technology gadget is part of the process, especially with cell phones and the dreaded 'Apps'. At no time in history has there been so much available to learn, and it been so easy to access. The internet and formal distance learning coupled with other on-line tools such as YouTube and Udemy means that today you can learn how to bake croissants or how to change the oil on your Toyota. Access and affordability have all shifted in the learner's favour.

The word "innovation" is derived from the Latin verb *innovare*, which means to renew, or to improve or to replace something, usually with something better than previously! But is there anything truly 'new' in the whole world? The real ground-breaking new stuff resides in the thousands of PhDs and other Doctorates written each year, but surely there is space here for us lesser mortals too. How do we innovate?

Well, for us it may be just doing something differently? Very many people get stuck doing the same things and getting the same mediocre or bad results. The stuck-in-a-rut place is a great place from which to innovate; it may take a minor touch on the steering wheel of life, or an almighty yank to find a new direction, but innovation will get you out. One thing is certain the wheels that created the original rut will at some point in the future create new ruts all over again, and the need to change again will emerge. Someone once said *"the only difference between a rut and a grave is the depth!"* Innovation, similar to learning is continuous as we hurtle through life.

In my own life, innovation has been key in developing ground-breaking new systems of communication. It was a simple as taking one working system and applying it to work over another already working system to produce a new and revolutionary one. In other ways, I used my military-acquired skillset as a basis to pivot into a variety of job sectors from the military to consultancy, to manufacturing key account management, to security industry director, to the health sector, and to being a non-fictional writer. I am left with only one question - what is next?

With my own optimistic life prognosis of another 20 years, I can surely fit in another change in the autumn of my years. If we apply the seasonal approach to life and innovation, then our early lives are full of "new stuff" but as we progress we become less and less inclined to innovate and change. I find it is important to keep this child-like enquiring mind and fearlessness in the face of the staid and unchangeable, and is vital if you want to innovate.

We must find our learning sources, as Ewald said, *"from every aspect of life",'* from each other, from reading, from looking, listening and from experiencing. Learning is a multi-dimensional and multi-sensory activity. Try and learn something new every day of your life!

Life Hack #1

Ask yourself - What season am I in? and what can I do differently today?

Often, we are most productive in the mind for new growth in the Autumn of our years! Many of the best business ideas came to those in their 60s. You're never too old for a good idea, often less work and more spare time, results in a huge innovative potential. Don't ever waste it!

Life Hack #2

Ask questions - for everything in life and especially in a confusing world filled with vast quantities of information and disinformation. Challenge everything with a child-like question and write down the answer. Challenge assumptions, as it is curiosity that fuels creativity. Someone says, *"Never" it* just means it's not been done yet!

Do not be conformed to this world, but be transformed by the renewal of your mind, that by testing you may discern what is the will of God, what is good and acceptable and perfect.

Romans 12:2

#2

Develop a sense of refreshment and energy

"There is nothing permanent except change."

Herodotus (c484BC-c425BC)
Greek historian.

"Order the steak rare. Eat an oyster. Have a negroni. Have two. Be open to a world where you may not understand or agree with the person next to you, but have a drink with them anyway."

Anthony Bourdain (1956-2018)
American celebrity chef, author, and travel documentarian.

"The reinvention of daily life means marching off the edge of our maps."

Bob Black (1951-present)
American musician, who played banjo in Bill Monroe's Blue Grass Boys.

I hope having just read the innovation wisdom you're ready to give it a try? But let's face it, you're never going to innovate sat on the sofa, in the same place, day after day. You need to continually opt to do thing differently in life and put your mind and body in different situations. By developing a sense of refreshment, this stimulates the mind and from the mind comes action, movement and personal development.

If we look to nature for guidance, we see many cycles. The earth's four equal seasons run in an annual cycle affecting all of the natural world. The 28-day lunar rhythm, effects the sea tides, animal migration & navigation, and the nocturnal behaviour of animals reliant on moonlight. Humans too have a natural rhythm driven by the day and night cycles of the Earth orbiting the Sun, called the circadian rhythm. We might also add the circle of life from birth to death, and for many the belief in rebirth and reincarnation when the soul returns again. The Law of Conservation of Energy states that "energy can neither created nor destroyed", energy can only change from one form into another. So, in the concept of our refreshment, we can only work with nature's numerous cycles and work to convert or enhance our energy levels.

In plant growth, for example, pruning is the best way to create growth, it is usually done in two ways. The first is a major cut-back in winter to remove damaged, diseased, and old wood in the plant's dormant phase. The aim of winter pruning is to promote vigour so that plants do not outgrow their space in the coming spring and summer seasons. Secondly, after the rush of spring growth and flowering, a final prune might be carried out to remove old flowers by deadheading and cutting back to the new buds, in an optimisation for full growth potential. Knowing what to cut out of your life, and when to do that can be a key catalyst to encouraging growth and that sense of refreshment.

Using the same metaphor, what fuel or fertiliser can we add for the growth we are trying to achieve? Do we go for fast, quick-fix off-the-shelf solutions or more organic ones aligned to nature; which type might be the best for you? Which has been around the longest? The key to sustainable growth, either in ourselves, nature or in organisations is that change agents themselves also have to change. Herodotus was quite correct when he said, *"There is nothing permanent except change."* Whatever is refreshing and reinvigorating changes you make now, might not always continue to work. We should keep mixing it up and continuously look for new sources in whatever we do, to pull new refreshing energy into our space.

Life Hack #1

Change the mundane! Changing your environment is like planting a bush in a new larger pot, giving it the space to grow! Changing the furniture layout of your room or house, try making new friends or relationships, trying new foods or hobbies can all create that same sense of newness and beginning that is so effective in helping you launch a new start. Be Anthony Bourdain for a few hours! Eat an oyster - maybe two?

Life Hack #2

Time to prune! Create space for the new stuff, clear the desk or clear out the wardrobe; just what is it cluttering-up your life right now. Do it today, it's either 'keep - rubbish - or charity shop'... at home or in your office space. You're already creating the potential space for new refreshing growth.

Come to me all you who are toiling and loaded down, and I will refresh you.

Matthew 11:28

#3

Beware of boredom

"Somebody's boring me.
I think it's me."

Dylan Thomas (1914-1953)
Welsh poet and writer whose works include poems and the "play for voices" Under Milk Wood.

"You need to let the little things that would ordinarily bore you suddenly thrill you."

Andy Warhol (1928-1987)
American artist, film director, and producer.

"Boredom is the dream bird that hatches the egg of experience.
A rustling in the leaves drives him away."

Walter Benjamin (1892-1940)
German Jewish philosopher, cultural critic, media theorist, and essayist.

To the French, it is called *'ennui'* or a feeling of listlessness and dissatisfaction arising from a lack of occupation or excitement, usually accompanied with lethargy. John Stott (1921-2011) the British Anglican priest once said, *"Apathy is the acceptance of the unacceptable."* Whichever description you chose, you know the feeling of being bored.

I am minded by the film title *Whose Life is it Anyway?* Well, it can only be your life, and if you're bored, it's your job to 'un-bore' yourself, much the same as being responsible for your own happiness. In later life I can well and truly recommend retirement - you'll never be busier, or so it would seem. But seriously, boredom is a state of mind stemming from either having nothing to do, having something to do and putting it off (procrastination) or having too much to do and being overwhelmed. Getting into too much of a routine or a rut and staying firmly in your comfort zone are the main ingredients for really a good self-indulgent boredom veg-out! Nothing wrong with that, once in a while - but it's not a lifestyle choice, is it? There are much better things to do, time to snap out of it.

Andy Warhol believed in finding excitement in everyday things, and often the mundane. He was responsible for the pop art movement in the 'swinging-sixties'. Warhol turned an image of a can of soup into a multi-million dollar work of art! How did he achieve that? You could say he put on a new pair of artistic glasses to 'see things differently'; he saw the potential in an ordinary boring mundane can of soup, to make it funky art. What do you see in your life that you can flip into something exciting?

In modern times, surely there is no excuse for being bored, but we often end up being bombarded with too much. Sit on your cell phone 'doom-scrolling' and suddenly you have wasted 2-hours, and achieved nothing. This is really next level hyper-boredom, a life flooded with boring meaningless things, time maybe to sort the 'wheat from the chaff.' This can be in your social life or at work and work boredom means it's time to make a change, be it revamp the office, hire some new staff or dust off the CV and change jobs.

Boredom, Ewald used to say *"is degeneration"* meaning one of decline or deterioration. It prevents our growth and keeps us in a closed loop, or a vicious circle, of doing nothing, thinking nothing, and improving nothing. The good news is, it's not a real illness and there are practical things to do, to snap out of it, and turn the vicious spiral of negativity into an improving virtuous one of positivity! Maybe, call your granny and ask her how her jam making is going this year? Or go cut the lawn or paint the kitchen ceiling you've been meaning to do for months... Oh my goodness! I hear you say - "I'm not that bored!"

Life Hack #1

Go to the Internet or better still an AI App and type in "your name - biography" and see what comes out. Better still type in a name of an old school friend you've often wondered about and see what pops up. You might even try a genealogical website and find a long-distant relative. Social reconnection can be an extremely interesting way to break boredom and discover new friends and may lead to a meeting or new adventure like a school reunion.

Life Hack #2

Try something new. Either a formal course or grab a YouTube video. I've always wanted to make my own sushi. I guess you've seen the price recently? Well, there are plenty of videos to watch to teach yourself how to make sushi and EVERYTHING else on the planet you've dreamed of ever doing is on the internet somewhere.

***Slothfulness casts into a deep sleep,
and an idle person will suffer hunger.***

Proverbs 19:15

#4

Adopt a state of oneness

"All differences in this world are of degree, and not of kind, because oneness is the secret of everything."

Swami Vivekananda (1863-1902)
Indian Hindu monk, philosopher, author, religious teacher, and the chief disciple of the Indian mystic Ramakrishna.

"Quantum physics thus reveals a basic oneness of the universe."

Erwin Schrodinger (1887-1961)
Austrian/Irish physicist who developed fundamental results in quantum theory, who won a Nobel Prize.

"The God who existed before any religion, counts on you to make the oneness of the human family known and celebrated."

Desmond Tutu (1931-2021)
South African Anglican Archbishop and theologian, known for his work as an anti-apartheid and human rights activist.

A state of oneness, paradoxically, can have several meanings in different dimensions. We could start with that basically *"Oneness is a unity with or part of someone or something,"*(Vocabulary.com) or *"a singleness of two things joined for a common state of being."* A married couple could achieve a oneness in their relationship, which makes it last for decades, 'till death do they part'. This is also a wonderful example, as oneness is not about achieving perfection, it allows for imperfection along the way, so long as the ultimate purpose is achieved. In my own marriage, my wife and I bicker over the smallest unimportant things imaginable, it drives our teenage son insane. It might be our coping mechanism, I'm not sure, but we've never had a really bad or regretful argument in over 20 years. We still live in a oneness, each making the other complete, although very far from perfect on the journey.

Oneness in nature might also be thought of as the circle of life, represented as birth, life, and death; and, for many, re-birth as the oneness of life continues in another spirit form. The oneness in this regard, overlaps from the mind into the soul, such that a oneness can be a sense of your own peace and connectedness within the universal realm some might call the divine. This inter-connectedness therefore transcends boundaries and dividers, as the heart-mind-centred feeling of being at one with the whole of the universe.

A true sense of oneness therefore requires a oneness in both thought and deed, and if that isn't an oxymoron, then I don't know what is! It is not enough to think of yourself as a kind human being, you actually have to translate that into action and do the kind acts in the real world. Oneness in purpose can translate into many dimensions and areas of our lives.

This new concept of oneness also fits with the ancient African philosophy of Ubuntu. Growing up as a young boy in the Eastern

Cape, Ewald must have been exposed to this and it resonated with him. Ubuntu or 'we are who we are because of others' fits with the notion that we are all connected to each other and nature in some unseen way. As Ewald said, *"To sum up the situation, is to realise that we are all part of a ONENESS and in contributing toward growth and evolution of the whole, we evolve and grow individually."*

Life Hack #1

Daily meditation or prayer can assist you in experiencing the interconnectedness of all the things in your life, seen and unseen. Quietening the mind, has proven benefits, even if only for a few minutes each day. Oneness starts in the mind, and then has to be translated into the actions of everyday life, which is the difficult part. Doing this is maybe all that is needed to connect your mind to everything else in your world, and the the World.

That they may all be one, just as you, Father, are in me, and I in you, that they also may be in us, so that the world may believe that you have sent me.

John 17:21

#5

My full potential self is the real me!

"Be yourself;
everyone else is already taken."

Oscar Wilde (1854-1900)
Irish poet and playwright.

"When you catch a glimpse of your potential,
that's when passion is born."

Zig Ziglar (1926-2012)
American author, salesman, and motivational speaker.

"The real question is, can you love the real me?
Not the perfect person you want me to be,
not that image you had of me,
but who I really am."

Christine Feehan (1999-present)
American paranormal romance novelist.

How do you achieve your full potential? First perhaps, you need to understand - who is the 'real you'? and to know that, you must know what is your purpose in life, ask yourself the question – Who am I? Hint: It is not that you're a doctor, or a wife, or own a house. You answer this by understanding your purpose in life and it's not a once-off question, it may change and in periods of your life change quite often! So maybe it is worth asking yourself annually. My purpose in life is...

Within your purpose is the real you and in meeting that purpose, why wouldn't you want to reach your fullest potential? But then perhaps, there is no full potential, perhaps, just perhaps it is unlimited in terms or size and unbounded in terms of scope, in all the various aspects of life. How much potential is enough?

As Ewald said, *"Imagine being in a peaceful place and at my fullest potential."* As always the answer lies within you, my 'fullest potential' I am sure will not be yours, and by-the-way, I intend never to limit my fullest potential. For me at least it's a contradiction in terms. So, in essence you'll never attain it, you just need to make peace with it in whatever period of your life you're in. Growth potential in terms of personal expectation can wax and wane as we move through life. Ambition may be a younger person's greatest asset, but just look at how many success stories there are of folk in later life, here are three.

The most famous is of Colonel Harland Sanders, who established the Kentucky Fried Chicken restaurant chain at 65. Nine years and 600 franchises later he sold his share for millions. In 2014, Yuichiro Miura, became the oldest person to reach the summit of Mount Everest at 80. Finally, Laura Ingalls Wilder, began writing "Little House on the Prairie" at 65; it later became a beloved television series. (Source: www.friendship.us/insights/).

It's never too late to go 'next-level potential', and in our later years we can be very productive indeed. I'm writing this at 66, already three books into my 10-book potential, but of course there may be more... One of the great enemies of your full potential is success, as this breeds a satisfying sense of complacency! My peaceful place is actually being on the journey, so long as I am moving forward in some mind, body and soul aspect I am happy. So pause, and take a well-deserved break when you're successful, but then do not rest for too long before restarting the journey. Setbacks and wrong turns are actually all part of the journey, and essential learning events, from which to gain your better and 'fuller potential.'

Life Hack #1

Read, read, read, and read some more! To grow we need stimulation and this often comes from a creative spark. Find good sources, and always exercise some discernment, especially with the internet, but try to read something every day, not limiting to one genre. Often, I'll go into a book shop (my ideas treasure house!) and pick up books on topics I've never even heard of, one of them gave me inspiration for the format for this book, before I had even conceptualised the draft.

Life Hack #2

Embrace what you view as 'failure or set-back'. Failure is a vital part of success, just ask JK Rowling ! She was turned down for her first Harry Potter book by every publishing house in the UK. Now that sounds familiar and in many ways I beat her in this regard, as my first military history book was turned down by every publishing house in the UK and South Africa. Although I sadly never reached her sales figures, I did not let failure deter me from my purpose. Next time you have a 'failure' write it down - ask yourself what did I learn? And what is my next step forward to improve?

The potential for every human being is great. Jesus wants you to live a highly productive life. He wants you to produce a crop - a hundred, sixty or thirty times what was sown.

Matthew 13:8

#6

Thinking is dangerous. Knowing is joy and pleasure

"There is nothing either good or bad but thinking makes it so."

William Shakespeare (c1564-1616)
English playwright, poet, and actor.

"To think too much is a disease."

Fyodor Dostoyevsky (1821-1881)
Russian novelist, and short-story writer.

"Man is a logical machine run by the scoundrels of emotions."

Raheel Farooq (Not Known)
Pakistani writer and spoken-word artist, who has created a keen interest in the ongoing dialogue between religion and science.

The premise is that; the act of thinking or processing some sort of data produces better answers than knowledge acquired over a long period of time. The application of knowledge over further time in various circumstances, leads to wisdom. Brian O'Driscoll, the famous Irish rugby player whimsically summarised this as *"Knowledge is knowing that a tomato is a fruit, wisdom is knowing not to put in a fruit salad."* Certainly true, but a quip he made to an interview made to avoid a penalty from a dressing room wager. He sounded wise for sure, but actually the 'wise answer' made no sense in the context of the question. Sadly, wisdom can only be acquired through the often-unsuccessful application of knowledge, and through many iterations. There are no short cuts in this regard.

Wisdom might also be considered intuition (gut-felt thinking), as opposed to logical (brain thinking) and emotional (heart-centered thinking). Each thinking centre plays its own part in the overall wisdom we acquire. But is it really the brain we need to take most care of in terms of how we apply it?, and it is not an 'age-thing' either. The traditional concept of the older you get the wiser you become, for sure applies to many people, but I've met very many young wise people too. It is more a state of mind, and some acquire that state much earlier than others, also some in their entire lifetime do not find their wise place.

For me at least - engineer's brain speaking now - thinking is not dangerous, as Ewald states, but for sure over-thinking at the wrong time can certainly be dangerous. A place of *"knowing"* and when in a state of *"joy and pleasure"*, is always a good place from which to think though, wouldn't you agree? The essence then to know what to do right now, rather apply the often fickle and indecisive brain to work it out for you. This comes from a place of knowledge and, to a degree experience, it is your inner truth.

Life Hack #1

Don't over-think situations and problems that require a decision, in the words of the Sport behemoth Nike® - *Just Do It.* If you're looking for ideas in odd places this is for sure one! The phrase was inspired by the final words of death row inmate Gary Gilmore who was due execution; who said, *"You know, let's do it."* The old adage that 'actions speak louder than words' is true, but I prefer when in doubt 'do something' and this usually comes from a place of knowledge and not over-thinking.

Life Hack #2

On the first day of my last posting in the British Army, while sitting at my desk in the Ministry of Defence, my boss, Barry said to me *"You really won't manage to do everything in this mad house, work out what you can achieve, the rest is most likely just noise."* He was quite correct too. Often there are tools such as the Pareto Rule (or the 80/20 Rule, where an 80% solution now can be better than a 100% solution way too late in the day. The rule, specifies that 80% of consequences come from about 20% of the causes, asserting an unequal relationship between inputs and outputs. So, make the 80/20 cut quickly - then *"Just Do It."*

To the Jews who believed him, Jesus said, If you hold to my teaching, you are really my disciples. Then you will know the truth, and the truth will set you free.

John 8:31-32

#7

Keep it simple!

"Life is really simple, but we insist on making it complicated."

Confucius (c551-c479 BCE)
Chinese philosopher and sage.

"Simplicity is the ultimate sophistication."

Leonardo da Vinci (1452-1519)
Italian polymath of the High Renaissance, painter, draughtsman, engineer, scientist, theorist, sculptor, and architect.

"Simple can be harder than complex. You have to work hard to get your thinking clean to make it simple. But it's worth it in the end because once you get there, you can move mountains."

Steve Jobs (1955-2011)
American businessman, inventor, investor, and co-founder of Apple Inc.

KISS! No, I don't want one, I'm good thanks... This is the accepted rule of 'Keep It Simple, Stupid', abbreviated to KISS. Another one I learned early in the Army. Plans made to be simple and easy to understand usually work better and quicker than overly complex ones. We live in an increasingly technological and complex world, where more and more, services, features, and 'things' are fed to us as must-haves on a daily basis. But do we really need them? Years ago, my Dad said, *"All I want from my cell phone is to call and speak to you."* Perhaps something to be respected from a generation who was responsible for the mobile phone and moon landings?

Ewald and Gail Meggersee were adamant in their teaching and application of the technique of BSR, that we are all 'enough'; so is the basic application of the technique quite enough. Nothing else was required, the basic technique they prescribed would, in most cases, assist the client perfectly well on their healing journey. The same applies to life, usually the simple approach works perfectly well, but due to various factors we have to add more and more to make it 'better'. Often thousands of man-hours of work went into making something simple that really works very well. Adding more, quite often, is far from better, it actually becomes worse. So we have to guard against over complicating matters, and just KISS it!

But why do we add detail when none is required? The first time I watched a PowerPoint presentation, when it was new out-of-the-box the presenter used every different animation for every different change to the presentation he could. It was a magnificent show, with words and images whizzing about in every direction. No one remembered what the presentation was about! That was 1987, since then I have only ever used two animation techniques for my slide shows. My second lesson, was learned during my Master's degree, 13 years later. My Telecommunications Module lecturer taught us for about 20 classes, where each class had at least 40 PowerPoint slides each crammed full of information. We were overwhelmed, so we asked him what we had to revise for the exams! His answer? *"Everything."* Needless to say, the majority of us scraped a pass.

But why do we do this? In the first instance my colleague wanted to impress, with the 'more is more concept' and which detracted from his overall message. In the second, my lecturer failed to distil and simplify into what was really important, probably resulting in less of an understanding of the whole topic. Most likely both were because of fear and/or insecurity. The last instance plays into the Steve Jobs quote, and that to get to the simple, required a great deal of time, effort and energy. Once you can do that in any situation, then you really can start to move mountains.

Life Hack #1

Relationships and connectedness are at the core of what do in life, so in exercising KISS or in 'keeping it real' there are two things I am sure you can improve on. The first is really listening by employing Active Listening to your interactions with others, by:

- Paying attention. Give the speaker your undivided attention, and be fully present and acknowledge the message...
- Showing that you are really listening...
- Providing feedback...
- Deferring judgment...
- Responding appropriately.

Life Hack #2

The second, following on from #1 is to 'say what you mean and mean what you say'. You have to talk your truth, be authentic, and say what it is you have to say. Then, we should have two people listening to understand and speaking to be understood. It is that simple?

There is no time to waste, so don't complicate your lives unnecessarily. Keep it simple, in marriage, grief, joy, whatever.

1 Corinthians 7:29-30

#8

Have an enquiring mind

"You only get answers to the questions you ask."

From the book
Good Leaders Ask Great Questions.

John C Maxwell (1947-present)
American author, speaker, and pastor who has written many books, primarily focusing on leadership.

"There are no foolish questions and no man becomes a fool until he has stopped asking questions."

Charles Proteus Steinmetz (1865-1923)
American mathematician, electrical engineer, and professor at Union College.

"No answer is also an answer."

Anon.

Having an enquiring mind is something we are born with; we are hardwired to be curious. It is part of our instinct and was a lifesaver to our ancestors. In fact, those who were most curious were used as the guards or sentries for danger, posted around settlements to watch for danger. Being intuitively curious was considered a special and highly valued skill. In many ways it still is, it most likely makes great innovators or inventors.

If you have had children, I am sure you will appreciate how toddlers rampage around the house, delving into every nook and cranny to find out what is there. Once they can speak then its *"Mum why...?"* twenty-four times a day. In case you didn't realise it, they are learning, and only what they want or need to get by. Often this changes when they get to school and it's time for institutionalised learning, then for some reason their enquiring mind can stop or at least malfunction somewhat. For those with 'straight-A' students, consider yourself blessed!

We are on a lifelong journey of learning, and having an enquiring mind is a really important skill. There is so much out there to enquire about and in case you didn't realise it, there is a competition to capture your attention, and especially so with the internet's 'click-baiting', where your enquiring mind is a target for some product marketeer! On-line, be focused and discerning with your inquisitiveness, try to find trusted sources, and remember these may not always be those you agree with all the time.

For many, asking questions can be difficult, it might seem like a sign of being stupid or a sign of weakness, and better not to expose yourself to this perception. But how else do you learn? The 'simplest, most basic question,' some will say, stupid question, gets every-one's attention because they wanted secretly to ask it but didn't! There are no stupid questions, only questions. Never stop having an enquiring mind, and of course all our minds enquire about different things at different times.

Life Hack #1

Enquiring Mind 101 - Ask Questions! They are the start point that fuel creativity and innovation. In making a decision or to try something new, ask yourself – What if I do it? Quickly followed by - what if I don't do anything?

Life Hack #2

Let go of the need to be right. Try to replace the need to be right in any situation with the desire to learn and acquire knowledge. This can open up the world of your belief system to a whole new set of options and opportunities. We learn best from each other, and in doing that try to learn from the best.

Instead of placidly accepting situations or scripture at face value, try asking the Holy Spirit to reveal new truths or change your perspective.

Deuteronomy 6:21

#9

We do not see the world as it is, but as we are

"We see the world, not as it is, but as we are or as we are conditioned to see it."

Stephen R Covey (1931-2012)
American educator, author, and businessman.

"When you look in the mirror, what do you see? Do you see the real you, or what you have been conditioned to believe is you? The two are so, so different. One is an infinite consciousness capable of being and creating whatever it chooses, the other is an illusion imprisoned by its own perceived and programmed limitations."

David Icke (1952-present)
English author, researcher, public speaker,
and a former footballer and sports broadcaster.

This means that the way we see things is a reflection of who we are or the world as a mirror. The original quote is credited to Anaïs Nin (1903-1977), a French-born American diarist, avant-garde novelist, and writer of short stories and erotica as, *"We see the world, not as it is, but as we are."* In this context we are both the observer, 'seeing' the world and also the participant 'being' a part of it. So, we see and filter the world, often rationalise it by our world view and the glasses through which we perceive it. Either an optimist views the world through 'rose-tinted spectacles' or negatively through 'black glasses'. The phrases both originate from Hebrew sayings. How do you see the world?

In the story the *Wizard of Oz*, anyone entering and living in the Emerald City had to wear a pair of emerald glasses, so that the citizens saw the city not as it was but as they saw it through the glasses. This means that people do not see the world objectively, but rather build a model or version of the world and impose that model on the rest of the world. As the book's author, L Frank Baum put it *"My people have been wearing green glasses on their eyes for so long that most of them think this really is an emerald city."* Maybe this sounds familiar in the current climate for, information, disinformation, and conspiracy theories? What glasses are you wearing?

If you want to change the world, is doing the same thing and getting the same bad outcome, then blaming the world or the environment, the best outcome? - then perhaps it's you who needs to change? Perhaps you need to change your glasses to get a different perspective? Or think about what Einstein said *"Doing the same thing over and over expecting a different result is insanity."* Time to change what you actually do as well.

In Stephen R Covey's version of the quote, he adds *"...as we are conditioned to see it."* Meaning that our world view although originating from our roots and upbringing is still shaped as we grow through life, and that there can be some manipulation or conditioning at play. We are conditioned by our work, family, religion, school, and society. We are taught from an early age, whom to be and how to think. Rather than being encouraged to find these things out for ourselves, we're taught to listen to what we're told. This listening leads to acting and this is how we are conditioned, rightly or wrongly.

Life Hack #1

Practise gratitude. What do you value and appreciate in life? Living a life in gratitude has many well-established benefits. It helps us to generate positive emotions, creates wonderful experiences, and fosters happy memories, all good for emotional health and well-being. Spend one week waking each day and writing down 5 different things you are grateful for.

Life Hack #2

Volunteer your time, talent or treasures. Studies have shown that where people give to charitable causes, or just to each other, they experience a sense of purpose and fulfilment. This can also have a positive impact on their mental health. Unconditional giving can help individuals put their own problems and concerns into perspective. In general, what 'you sow, you reap' and the world as a mirror, returns to you manyfold. You may not have much to give, but that's not the point, finding the place to give comes from the heart and not always the wallet. Find your place(s) to give...

Life Hack #3

Journaling! At the end of the day spend just 5 minutes reflecting on the world and write down your thoughts. How did you treat the world and how did it treat you back? You will always be work-in-progress, so some positive and negative thoughts are always acceptable. Introspection will create awareness, from which you can learn for the next similar interaction.

Anyone who listens to the word but does not do what it says is like someone who looks at his face in a mirror and, after looking at himself, goes away and immediately forgets what he looks like.

James 1:23-24

#10

The World as abundance

"If you want love and abundance in your life, give it away."

Mark Twain (1835-1910)
American writer, humourist, and essayist Samuel L Clemens used the pen name Mark Twain.

"When you undervalue who you are, the world will undervalue what you do and vice versa."

Suze Orman (1951-present)
American financial advisor, author, and podcast host.

"Shoot for the Moon. Even if you miss, you'll land among the stars."

Norman Vincent Peale (1898-1993)
American clergyman, author best known for popularising the concept of positive thinking.

Fortunately, as large-brained entities at the top of the food chain we have knowledge, experience, and emotion, but unfortunately, we're born with an awareness that we are going to die. It's an in-built scarcity limiting factor, and the realisation that we only have 'three score years and ten' or about 70-years, to do what we have to do in life. We are programmed to be finite, after birth, the only surety is death. This in-built fear drives us to save money, own property, buy insurance, even though they are considered the norm and 'wise'. Modernity preys on this and fuels the scarcity fear we are born with. Watch the news, (funny we used to say 'read the news'); it's mainly, famine, drought, job loss, high cost of living, cutbacks, scarcity of money. Yet, in any one moment, life is abundant, how so I hear you say...?

Let's do the obvious one – money! I guess you could do with a little more? Guess what? You have never been richer and you mostly likely place in the top 5% richest people in the World if you bought my book! A wealth programme in the UK said, *"If you have a small dish in your house where you drop your loose change - you're in the top 5% richest people in the World."* Yes, it means the vast majority are really that poor, one billion people live on less than $1.00 per day and 46%, or 3,5 billion people live on $5.50 per day or less. How much was your last latté? I'll tell you, in 2025, it's around $5.46 for the American national average latté!

Perhaps, consider that wealth is a continuously flowing river and not a finite cake to be divided up, there is an abundance of money, it is maybe not in the right place, at the right time to meet your needs? Living in abundance, means having a prosperity and abundance mindset. In setting up BSR practices for his new students, Ewald would always preach, *"Worry about the thousands you will have to turn away..."* What a mindset, and it all starts with intention, and intentions can be dreams, so DREAM BIG and

"Shoot for the Moon" and, if you miss?, among the stars is not a bad place to end up!

Life Hack #1

This is simple - give away something you really treasure and see what happens! Wow, this one is scary for sure and remember you have time, talent, and treasures. The act of giving is both fulfilling in itself, and it often leaves space for the world to abundantly fill it with something much better...

Life Hack #2

Actively celebrate in other's success. In this way, you can trigger self-acceptance that positively impacts your self-worth. With a habit of praising others, it's only a matter of time before you start accepting and praising yourself, and you can also share in other's success and wins. If you are in a state of appreciation, and not envy or competition, other abundance will rub off on you.

The thief comes only to steal and kill and destroy; I came that they may have life and have it abundantly.

John 10:10

#11

Don't fix what is wrong, work on what's right

"Life is too short to talk about the small, unimportant things when you catch the bigger picture."

Mya (1979-present)
American singer, songwriter, dancer, record producer, and actress.

"Do what is right, not what is easy nor what is popular."

Roy T Bennett (Not Known)
American author of The Light in the Heart, who shares positive thoughts and creative insights that has helped people to live a successful and fulfilling life.

"If you are working on something that you really care about, you don't have to be pushed. The vision pulls you."

Steve Jobs (1955-2011)
American businessman, inventor, investor, and co-founder of Apple Inc.

Often the news in today's media is all about negative and wrong things, which tend to be a minority of world events, while most of the world really is pretty good. Unfortunately, in our human psyche it has to be said, good is un-newsworthy. Psychologically, we are more triggered by negative news than positive news, we simply pay more attention to seemingly 'bad news' than good news. Humans have an in-built negativity bias, its hard-wired into us, as part of the scarcity factor. It refers to our disposition to 'attend to, learn from, and use negative information far more than positive information' (Vaish, Grossmann, & Woodward, 2008). This means we're prone to fix things and spend so much time doing it we fail to attend to improving what we're are already doing correctly, those good things Ewald refers to.

Mainstream western medicine's focus is to fix what's wrong piecemeal... but not work on the whole body (what's generally right). Fixing the smaller things that are wrong will fail to attend to what is required by way of maintenance for the whole body.

In Ewald and Gail's discovery of BSR, through its application on Ewald, the whole was certainly more important that the small and painful parts. As soon as the focus for them shifted towards the less painful and 'more right whole' - the secrets of the modality were unlocked.

Life Hack #1

Focus on what is going well in your life at the moment, one topic for a day. Write down and write 5 statements to accompany each one to say how you might improve it or do it better. Do this for seven days; repeat when the 'bad news' start to get at you again.

Life Hack #2

Ask for feedback in those seven areas you've just worked on. It might be your clients or customers, family members, your best friend or your students. You might create an amazing list of client testimonials, even better you'll build self-confidence and self-esteem for all the amazing achievements you're getting right. Note to self - expect some criticism on the way, life's not perfect, correct it, and move on.

So, we fix our eyes not on what is seen, but on what is unseen, since what is seen is temporary, but what is unseen is eternal.

2 Corinthians 4:18

#12

Make the effort to become effortless

"Logically, somebody who never put effort into anything should be the master of effortlessness. But it is not so. If you want to know effortlessness, you need to know effort. When you reach the peak of effort, you become effortless."

Sadhguru (1957-present)
Indian guru and founder of the Isha Centre in Coimbatore, India.

"Past a certain point, more effort doesn't produce better performance. It sabotages our performance. Economists call this the law of diminishing returns."

Greg McKeown (1977-present)
American author, public speaker, leadership and business strategist.

Did you ever watch David Beckham take free kicks? The term "Bend it like Beckham" became a buzzword for the mastery of a particular skill. The physics of doing that by the way is called the Magnus Effect. Striking the ball off-centre changes the pressure dynamic on one side by spinning the ball and makes it turn in the air. He did it with some natural talent, but then added countless hours of practice. Once team training was finished, he used to take over 50 practice free kicks, building up hours of skill and muscle memory. He scored over 65 free kicks in his career, ranking number 6 on the world's all-time greatest list. He became truly effortless and scored some amazing free kicks for Manchester United, and England.

It takes effort, more than that actually, real hard, time-consuming gruelling toil at times, to be the best you can at what you do. You may not be training to be the world champion at something, but finding that place of effortlessness in your work or sport can bring incredible joy. Those world champions are working harder than all of their peers, it is what they have to do to get to the top in their competitive field. For the rest of us, there is no substitute for doing the work, and a little improvement often is all that is needed. Have you heard of the "1% Rule?"

The 1% Rule by Tommy Baker, the business entrepreneur, and author of the *1% Rule: How to Fall in Love with the Process and Achieve your Wildest Dreams*, states *"that if you consistently and persistently be better at what you do by 1% each day, that over the course of 100-days, you will be 100% better."*(Summaries.com). It works on micro-progress, and very similar to the compound effect usually associated with savings. It adds progress on progress, so that each day you're starting from a new improved base. Of course it sounds easy, but takes a great deal of effort to create a small change that will stick today and not need effort on it tomorrow, as tomorrow there is another change coming! The key is to strive for very small, improvements, you might hardly notice them in terms of time and effort, but it does provide an overall improvement.

Life Hack #1

Prioritise on what is crucial and focus on it relentlessly. Plan and set time aside for it, cut out the distractions, wake-up earlier, and do it more often. One day you'll be in the middle of doing it, and you won't even know it. Now you are effortless.

Life Hack #2

Get up one hour early! In that one hour, there is time for plenty, 1-cup of coffee, 10-minutes meditation and to create that 1% improvement you need to find. There will even some time left over to add another valuable life hack. Even if you just do this on week days – that's 260-hours of improvements you can make in 1 year. Such is the 'Power of One'. In maths any number raised to the power of "1" equals itself. It is the power of singularity, one idea at a time, focus on one change with total presence and thought, to stand the best chance of success.

"Whatever you do, work heartily, as for the Lord and not for men."

Colossians 3:23

#13

Emotions bring the largest discord to humanity

"Anger is never without a reason, but seldom a good one."

Benjamin Franklin (1706-1790)
American writer, scientist, inventor, statesman, Freemason, diplomat, printer, publisher, and political philosopher.

"I've learned that people will forget what you said, people will forget what you did, but people will never forget how you made them feel."

Maya Angelou (1928-2014)
American memoirist, poet and, civil rights activist.

"I don't want to be at the mercy of my emotions. I want to use them, to enjoy them, and to dominate them."

From A Portrait of Dorian Gray.

Oscar Wilde (1854-1900)
Irish poet, and playwright.

Emotions are the Yin or Yang, the left or right, and the black or white of how we chose to interact with the world around us. In common belief, they are centred in the heart where love resides right next to its ugly opposite - hatred. Being 'heart-centred' is good and meaningful, but also be cognisant of the intuitive gut and the thinking mind. "The Perfect You" or its version at any time, and how you interact with the World is key - in how the World interacts with you. Ewald used to say *"Emotions bring disagreement"*, perhaps because they are fickle and there is always the ugly flip-side waiting to emerge. Many people are, of course prone to the flip side, ugly emotions, negative feelings, and wrong actions more of the time than good ones. The World perhaps is most significantly represented to us through the mainly negative media, as this most appeals to us. We are more and more called on be emotional and shocked and offended, and to suspend our discernment and intelligence in making value judgements. Ewald also taught in his BSR Principles Class *"I am perfect."*

As we can train the mind to gain intelligence and have a high IQ, or Intelligence Quotient so we can similarly train our emotions through an EQ or Emotional Quotient. The term first appeared in 1965, but this measure become hugely popular in 1995 with author Daniel Goleman, and his best seller *Emotional Intelligence*. Well worth a read if you're prone to interacting with the world solely based on emotions.

In my BSR practice, I see many suffering from emotional stress, which usually manifests in the shoulders, neck and head. We have a natural but subtle tendency to permanently hunch our shoulders, when suffering from emotional stress, often resulting in headaches, reduced neck motion and tight neck muscles. Some I feel are more prone to it than others, and 'leading with emotions' is never a good idea. Are your own emotions bringing you discord in your personal world, or can you filter out the flip-side emotions and lead with more emotional intelligence?

Life Hack #1

All it takes is one breath. Next time you feel stressed, or angry or about to explode, all you have to do is take one deep, and I mean really deep single breath. Four seconds in, hold it slightly, and four seconds out. Breathe in and out through the nose for optimum oxygen intake. The pause is usually all you need to calm the heart and mind. Now you're ready to respond from a position of calm.

Life Hack #2

Stick to the high ground. When Michelle Obama said, *"When they go low, we go high"*, it meant to not sink to the lowest common denominator. Apply this to all you do, emotionally intelligent leaders, apply decorum and take the 'high road', meaning they refuse to sink below their ethical standards. It is not always the easiest path to take, but going on the low road, is to take an ethical or moral short cut, and has no possible pay-off.

But don't let the passion of your emotions lead you to sin!

Ephesians 4:26

#14

Where the mind is focused, energy flows

"Energy flows where attention goes. To get what you really want in life, you need a clear goal that has purpose and meaning behind it. Once this is in place, you can focus your energy on the goal and become obsessive about it. When you learn how to focus your energy, amazing things happen."

Antony Jay Robbins (1960-present)
American author, coach, and speaker.

"Focus on being productive instead of busy."

Tim Ferriss (1977-present)
American entrepreneur, investor, author, podcaster, and lifestyle guru.

"One way to boost our willpower and focus, is to manage our distractions instead of letting them manage us."

Daniel Goleman (1946-present)
American psychologist, author, and science journalist.

As Ewald used to say about starting up a BSR practice, *"Where attention goes, energy flows; where energy flows, capacity grows."* This is the principle of intent, and having intention is the first step to change and growth. Of course, Ewald was talking about the focus of practitioner to client in that moment of applying the BSR technique. It equally applies to every-thing else you do in life.

The full quote by Tony Robbins however gives us a fuller picture of the mind-focus development idea. To be effective in life you need to start with something at the top, a life goal, a vision or a purpose. Yes, we're back to purpose - AGAIN! The mind is flighty, too much to do, too little time to fit in everything. Most of us need 28 hours in a day to fit ordinary things in, and it's a day the geyser didn't burst - yet. Keeping a day on-track, on-message and on-purpose, can be hard work, very hard work. Ever get to lunch time and wonder *"What on earth have I achieved this morning?"*

While our subconscious mind is running the show and all our life sustaining activities, it still leaves unimaginable computing power, with which to do our mind-focusing thing. Let's face it, focusing on something doesn't stop us digesting food and carrying out all the other body functions. Nope, the 5% conscious mind is more than enough for you, just that everyone else would also like to grab its attention too. Who needs a piece of you? Trivia at work, spouse needs some 'me-time', then every call centre and ad agency in the world is hunting you too on every possible media platform you can imagine.

It is easy to be busy, not so easy to be productive. The brain has a way of avoiding the important difficult on-purpose stuff. It creates something else equally as important and much more fun that really needs doing instead, like tidying-up all the paper clips in the office drawer. It is called procrastination... distractions are a way to ignore or put off the real-deal business. It is a self-sabotaging activity that gives you a quick fix, then you've wasted time, and you feel guilty about it.

Life Hack #1

What are you putting off? What is currently on the 'To Do' List? My problem is I usually have too many lists and each one has way too many tasks on it. Maybe it is best to consolidate all your lists onto one daily list? Have two or three 'MUST-DOs' and then some 'NICE-TO-DOs' later. Hint: Always do the 'MUST-DOs' first!

Life Hack #2

Being productive - the Pareto Principle works here... focus on the core 20% of important tasks to achieve your purpose or goal - the rest is 'fluff'. Some things just don't need to be done or done by you specifically. Deferral or delegation is a great way to try and focus on what you need to. Don't take on other's 'To Do' lists, they are not yours to do!

Let your eyes look straight ahead;
fix your gaze directly before you.

Proverbs 4:25

#15

Be Open

"People are very open-minded about new things, as long as they're exactly like the old ones."

Charles Kettering (1876-1958)
American inventor, engineer, businessman, and the holder of 186 patents.

"A mind is like a parachute. It doesn't work if it is not open."

Frank Zappa (1940-1993)
American musician, composer, and bandleader.

"What the world needs most is openness: Open hearts, open doors, open eyes, open minds, open ears, open souls."

Robert Mueller (1944-present)
American lawyer who served as the sixth director of the Federal Bureau of Investigation from 2001 to 2013.

We are still in the mind domain, so openness here relates to the mind, meaning that openness is *"the quality of being willing to consider ideas and opinions that are new or different to your own"* (Cambridge Dictionary). Or *"An open mind means one free of bias and unhealthy mental models. To be mindful is to be consciously aware, objectively seeing things as they are, moment to moment."* (ProjectManagement.com).

This, in a whole-body context, also allows our bodies to be 'open' to try and experience new ways of healing itself. A state that our clients in BSR find helps them to accept that the new modality they experience will actually work. There is even a hashtag for it; #BSRWorks. Just because something is different to the traditional does not mean it won't work, it just means you've not tried it or experienced it yet. We see many clients at the end of a long journey through mainstream western medicine where it didn't quite work out for them. Conversely, rarely do we see the ones where it did work. Both have their place in the health and well-being sector, and the BSR technique works in a complementary way to the mainstream, and not something different or competing with it.

Ewald certainly did have some very open and different views on mainstream medicine, and was very open to all ideas and concepts regarding it. He was after all a trained medical doctor of chiropractic, and more qualified than me to debate these 'other views'. While I am open-minded, I don't feel qualified to represent his views or debate them here, nor do they fit my world view as a BSR practitioner, whereby we stay in our lane and do not criticise or represent medical opinions to our clients. In your own openness, you will have to decide for yourself what you accept into your world view, and, let's face it there is a great deal of opinion coming our way these days on YouTube, Tik Tok, and every other information source, even in university research papers. In assessing what to allow credence to in your own world view, I always start with - what is the writer's motivation for writing this piece, for whom do they work, and what is the platform style? I hope I explained my own motivations well enough at the beginning of the book, and you understand my world view?

Being open-minded means having empathy to understand and consider another's view or perspective, even if you disagree with them. Understand the place they are coming from, as it is what motivates their world view and decisions. COVID-19 and the 'vaccinate or not to vaccinate' debate is a case in point. During the pandemic, in the first wave, my wife lost 10 relatives and in the second wave another 5 in her extended African family. Our family vaccinated and boosted once; our world view was influenced by our experiences. Others had a totally different view and experience, and maybe had relatives they believed died of the vaccine, but we may never know the truth. Either way, it was a personal decision and I respect it, that is what being open is all about.

Of course, it doesn't mean that there are no limits, or 'guard-rails' to understanding the other person's view, you don't have to have empathy for every ideology under the sun. After the Charlotteville clash in America between a Black Lives Matter march and an white supremacist faction, The President, Donald J Trump remarked *"There are very fine people on both sides."* I give you, he may have meant in a wider political debate on the monuments that still exists to the Confederacy in the Deep South, but the words still give room to empathise with racism. Is it what you would want to do in your own openness? So take care exactly what you chose to align or empathise with, have your own guard rails for your own world view protection. As Ewald often said *"Don't back yourself into a corner,"* and some corners are just really best avoided.

Life Hack #1

Connect with people who have a variety of perspectives or a different perspective to you. Right now, I have someone who is really getting under my skin, he is very different to me, but I have to find a way understand him and his world view. In being open to their ideas, I can grow my own understanding, and maybe pull myself out of my own corner, and back into a more open and creative space. Who is that person in your life? Try to connect and listen to them, and understand their perspective, for sure it is going to be difficult but will also grow you.

Life Hack #2

Explore! No need to sign-up and climb in the Himalayas - I bet there is somewhere local - a museum or building, a suburb or park - you've never been to before and always wondered about. Time to visit, and see what you can find, be open to being wrong. I live in South Africa, crime is all over, I have to take care when I metal detect. In my exploration, I metal detect in my local parks. So far, I've met one of my ardent Facebook followers, a preacher with an interesting life story and Joshua who always wanted to be an architect, but instead builds his own guest houses. So far, fingers crossed or as 'Saffas' say, holding thumbs - I've not been mugged!

We should be moving toward openness with each other, trusting that our brothers and sisters love us and will help us.

1 John 1:7

#16

Ego alert!

"Check your ego at the door. The ego can be the great success inhibitor. It can kill opportunities, and it can kill success."

Dwayne 'The Rock' Johnson (1972-present)
American actor, professional wrestler, and businessman.

"Your ego can become an obstacle to your work. If you start believing in your greatness, it is the death of your creativity."

Marina Abramovic (1946-present)
Serbian conceptual and performance artist, her work explores body art and endurance art.

"It takes humility to seek feedback. It takes wisdom to understand it, analyse it and appropriately act on it."

Stephen R Covey (1931-2012)
American educator, author, and businessman.

This wisdom very much leads on from being open-minded, and stems from the desire to place yourself before others. It is about your self-esteem and self-importance and striking the balance. It may be fine to have a good view of your own self-esteem or value to the world, but wholly wrong to allow that to become an importance of self over others. Then you are in the realms of ego and placing your views and worth at a higher value than others.

But if we are open-minded, where might ego be an asset? One case that springs to mind is Mohammad Ali. Who can doubt that he truly was *"The Greatest"* when he walked in a room he would even declare *"The Champ is here!"* He used ego and bravado, as a strategy against his opponent, making himself to believe he'd already won before even entering the boxing ring. Of course, he was a great showman and many times his opponents most likely thought they were going to lose too. In a real fight of this nature, you might use a little ego, or let's call it 'overt self-esteem' to get the edge. In the words of Ali, *"It's hard to be humble when you're as great as I am."* Who can argue with that? and the world loved him for it. Outside the ring and in later life however, he was a humble and well-respected man. All just a show, and not genuine ego.

The danger is when you're not in a fight as he was, and just in a space where you believe you know more, and are better in some way than any one of the other 8 billion people on the planet. You really are not. In our journey of growth to being the best version of ourselves, it never means we have to take away from others to achieve that. Being egotistical and tearing another person down, does not add to your worth in any way. The true leaders in life will always seek to be better by empowering others and building strong teams. It was Sir Ken Robinson, the bestselling author, who said, *"What you do for yourself dies with you when you leave this world, what you do for others' lives on forever."* This attitude and behaviour rarely comes from a place of ego. One of my greatest joys in the military was losing a valued member of the team as they were promoted and posted off to a new unit, always sad to see them go but proud of having been a small part of their success. It's okay to feel a little pride now and then, but never let it turn to ego.

Life Hack #1

Stop comparing yourself to others, it's an ego thing and the ego is looking for validation. Comparing past to present can always leave us falling short, and our ego will punish us and effect our self-worth. You are already good enough and unique and incomparable to anyone else. By stopping this activity, we shift the focus back to our own consciousness, and humility, to be the best version of ourselves, without the need to measure against someone else. My author best buddy told me how many books he'd sold once, it was over 20 000, I immediately compared it to my meagre 1200 books, when I really should not have, well I did ask him - my big mistake. I really am content with my own success, without comparison.

Life Hack #2

Stop complaining. Constant negativity is the source from where self-loathing and self-sabotage comes from, and our ego feeds off it. Usually it says *"See I told you, you weren't good enough."* Stop complaining for a week, or maybe a month. Every time you think you might moan even a little, return to being grateful for the positive things in your life, see what this opens up for you.

Life Hack #3

Ask for advice. It takes humility to ask for advice, and sometimes even greater humility to receive feedback, but you send a message to the world that you want to grow. Everyone needs a little help now and then - even you.

Pride goes before destruction,
a haughty spirit before a fall.

Proverbs 16:18

#17

'Allowingness'

"Something amazing happens when we surrender and just love. We melt into another world, a realm of power already within us. The world changes when we change. The world softens when we soften. The world loves us when we choose to love the world."

Marianne Williamson (1952-present)
American author, speaker, and political activist.

"You are afraid of surrender because you don't want to lose control. But you never had control; all you had was anxiety."

Elizabeth Gilbert (1969-present)
American journalist and author.

"Whatever comes, let it come, what stays let stay, what goes let go."

Hariwansh Lal Poonja or 'Papaji' (1910-1997)
Indian Hindu sage.

'Allowingness' is a powerful concept by which you act and then step back and let things be and flow from that action. In many situations we act and then fiddle, and over control, which is often counterproductive. The Control Freak is going to find this a difficult concept to grasp. There is often a trust or self-confidence element to this notion too, 'allowing' also means to trust in the process you're applying or in your own skill or abilities. Self-doubt and allowingness are not good bed-fellows! Being in control can be something of a drug, the more we do it the more we want to control other aspects which are entirely out of our reach. But how much are we in control? Did you know that only 5% of our brain's activity is conscious thought while the other 95% is subconscious. Take that, Control Freak! This means that the majority of the decisions, actions, and emotions we have in a day are coming from the part of the brain that lies beyond our conscious awareness. We're virtually in a state of allowingness already, just obsessing over 5% of what we are aware of. Your mind surrendered control to a part of your brain, you don't really have access to anymore.

Allowingness, also has a time and space element, and in that act of literally stepping-back, it gives these two potent factors the opportunity to act. This concept for healing most BSR practitioners see on their client's healing journey quite frequently, 'Time being that great healer'. Space and absence also provide an opportunity for growth and change, and often finding uncluttered physical spaces in nature gives our brain the opportunity to free-wheel, heal, and be creative.

A good example of this was when Gail and Ewald were heading towards literally their last packet of food while studying in America. Gail the ever practical was worried about how they were going to eat, while Ewald was prepared to allow for the prospect of nothing. Allowing, trusting, and knowing fell into place as two friends offered them jobs the very next day. Allowingness and absence gave the space needed for something to be provided.

Similarly, with the three tenets of this book of mind, body, and soul, being completely connected and interdependent in the wider world, connectedness is important for 'allowingness to fully work. Much as it is difficult to 'just be' in modern society, we are, as the human race always interconnected. For Ewald, Ubuntu, must have completely spoken to his allowingness belief. Ubuntu or *"we are who we are because of others"* or *"Allow others to just be, as you would wish to be."* Ewald was a fan of Credo Mutwa (1921-2020) who was a renowned South Africa author and traditional healer who wrote the book, *Indaba, My Children*. In the book, Mutwa shares his deep understanding of African spirituality, mythology, and cultural heritage. Allowingness is a central theme to these elements of African Philosophy.

Life Hack #1

In creating space; less can definitely be more. Old clothes need to go, the garage needs a de-clutter, the pantry and old food tins just have to go, and take a look at your workspace. Making physical clean space also frees the mind too and puts us in a better state for allowingness to really happen.

Life Hack #2

Letting go of control, the Control Freak is already thinking of how to skip this one! So let's make it easy, and not ask you to do something, but to stop doing something. Our words create our reality, so changing how we phrase our environment can reduce the urge to control, try these shifts in the words you use:

From *"You must try this!"* to *"Have you ever considered trying this?"*
From *"The problem is…."* To *"Maybe this difficulty is an opportunity to change…"*
From *"You must do it this way…"* to *"Is there a better way?"*
From *"I'll check on you tomorrow…"* to *"Come back to me when you're finished."*
From *"I'll do it"* to *"Please will you do this…"*

Life Hack #3

Now that you know you're not in control, it's time to reprogramme that subconscious mind, and it really can be done over time. There are lots of ways, but here is one that operates contrary to our society and news media! Spend the day with not one single negative thought. When you're about to have one - quickly replace it with a different one. Here's an example of how to alter perspective:

Negative: *"I'm not good enough to get promoted."*
Replace with the positive: *"I am continually improving my skills and gaining in experience, I am on the right path."*

Once you've done one 100% positive day - try another and another….

Thou shalt love thy neighbour as thyself.

Matthew 22:37-39

#18

Never judge others

"Mindfulness means moment-to-moment, non-judgmental awareness. It is cultivated by refining our capacity to pay attention, intentionally, in the present moment, and then sustaining that attention over time as best we can. In the process, we become more in touch with our life as it is unfolding."

Jon Kabat-Zinn (1944-present)
American professor emeritus of medicine and the creator of the Stress Reduction Clinic and the Center for Mindfulness in Medicine.

"I find hope in the darkest of days, and focus in the brightest." I do not judge the universe."

14th and current Dali Lama (1935-present)
Tibetan spiritual leader and head of Tibetan Buddhism.

"Instead of putting others in their place, put yourself in their place."

Amish Proverb.

No coincidence I meet you here, you've recently come from the ego wisdom right? Which always uses the judgment to get the worst out of you in making you feel superior; or in making you feel bad by not being good enough. Time to stop being judgemental, as opposed to a few judgements here and there. But what is the difference?

At the purest level, we make decisions by judgement, the continual measurement of where we are against our own set of beliefs, values, and needs. In this regard, judgement is an important and positive part of self-development as we follow our purpose and life-plan. It becomes bad when we are judgemental of others, setting up our own standards and 'moral high ground' to be better than that of someone else. This is when we set up our standard to be the best and measure others against it, believing ourselves superior in some way. Now we're being judgemental.

In modern society we are constantly judged, and asked to judge others. Judging can be a marketing strategy. Look at this - judge - be horrified - and click on the story. But how can we avoid ever being judgemental of others?

Jon Kabat-Zinn sums it up well as that *"Mindfulness means moment-to-moment, non-judgemental awareness"* Meaning we have to stay very present in the day-to-day moments we are faced with and to be in a state of mindfulness. This is *"a mental state achieved by focusing one's awareness on the present moment, while calmly acknowledging and accepting one's feelings, thoughts, and bodily sensations used as a therapeutic technique."*
(Oxford Dictionary).

Life Hack #1

When you find yourself about to judge someone, ask yourself *"But what do I really know about them."* You, me, everyone has a history and some baggage, right? Do you know mine? Well of course I'm not about to tell you, and the person you're about to judge, surely won't be telling you theirs either. Maybe if we all knew each other's baggage then we might be less judgemental? Someone recently told me theirs in the heat of a disagreement, and guess what, it really helped me understand their point-of-view much better. We still disagree, but maybe with a touch more humanity, and I'm a lot less judgemental on why they behave the way they do.

Life Hack #2

I am sure you have heard the saying *"Don't judge someone unless you've walked a mile in their shoes,"* which is the same concept as the Amish quote previously. Put yourself in their place, maybe not literally in their shoes, but just imagine if it were you walking alongside them, experiencing and feeling the same they were, but in a parallel way. Imagine or better still empathise how you would feel and cope. Understand their situation, it maybe you one day, savour that thought.

Do not judge, or you too will be judged.

Mathew 7:1

#19

Let Intuition 'sneak in'

"It turns out that our intuition is a greater genius than we are."

Jim Shepard (1956-present)
American novelist, and short-story writer.

"Intuition will tell the thinking mind where to look next."

Jonas Salk (1914-1995)
American virologist and medical researcher who developed one of the first successful polio vaccines.

"You have to leave the city of your comfort and go into the wilderness of your intuition. What you'll discover will be wonderful. What you'll discover is yourself."

Alan Alda (1936-present)
American actor, best known for playing Captain "Hawkeye" Pierce in the wartime sitcom M*A*S*H.

The definition of intuition is: *"Knowledge from an ability to understand or know something immediately based on your feeling,* (often referred to as a 'gut-feeling'), *rather than facts."* Or *"an ability to understand or know something without needing to think about it or use reason to discover it."* (www.wholesomeculture.com/)

Much like the reflex action we have when touching a hot stove and immediately pulling our hand away without thinking about it – so our 'gut-feeling' is our immediate response feeling, it tells us the right thing to do. Intuition acts like the guardian of what is right or best, it takes the brain's logic and the heart's emotions to craft wisdom. The problem is many people do not empower their intuition and prefer to logically reason and process facts to come up with a 'better version' or answer, but which often leads to the wrong outcome!

When either the heart's emotional decisions or the brain's processed logic gets it wrong, who's there to put you right – good ol' Mr Intuition who says, *"I told you so!"* You knew what was right and proper to do all along, but reasoned to do it differently anyway, and your way.

Intuition really is your inner genius, some you might argue garnered from nature in our 'caveman' genes and some perhaps from nurture, how we were raised with societal norms etc. Either way a life where intuition is more often allowed to "sneak in" and tapped into, may be a life lived more wisely, or as Ewald used to say *"Trust the gut."* In fact, better than letting it sneak in, ask the gut straight way, and listen to the immediate answer. The answer is like an 'intuitive reflex', it comes without thinking from the brain, or without the heart's emotions. Get it? - got it? - good, it has to be that quick!

Life Hack #1

What should you do when facing tricky choices?
Ask yourself the question, *"Should I do or chose X...?"* (Only one thing, not two)
Then immediately tap into your inner gut-feeling; and say, *"Does that feel heavy or light?"*
Heavy = wrong and light = right.
And don't wait, because then your brain starts to think and process, and say, *"Feels heavy for sure BUT... we can do it this way instead."*

Life Hack #2

Try Automatic Writing. This is the process or free writing or writing what first comes into your head, for any given scenario, without thinking it through. Otherwise known as tapping into your sub-conscious brain, which we now know controls 95% of your life! Often the answer may lay somewhere in there.

Life Hack #3

Practices such as deep purposeful breathing, meditation or walks outside in the fresh air are not just healthy; they also sharpen our ability to connect with your gut-feelings. These activities can be easily integrated into any routine, clear your mind and create a space where your inner voice becomes clearer and stronger.

The way of a fool is right in his own eyes,
but a wise man listens to advice.

Proverbs 12:15

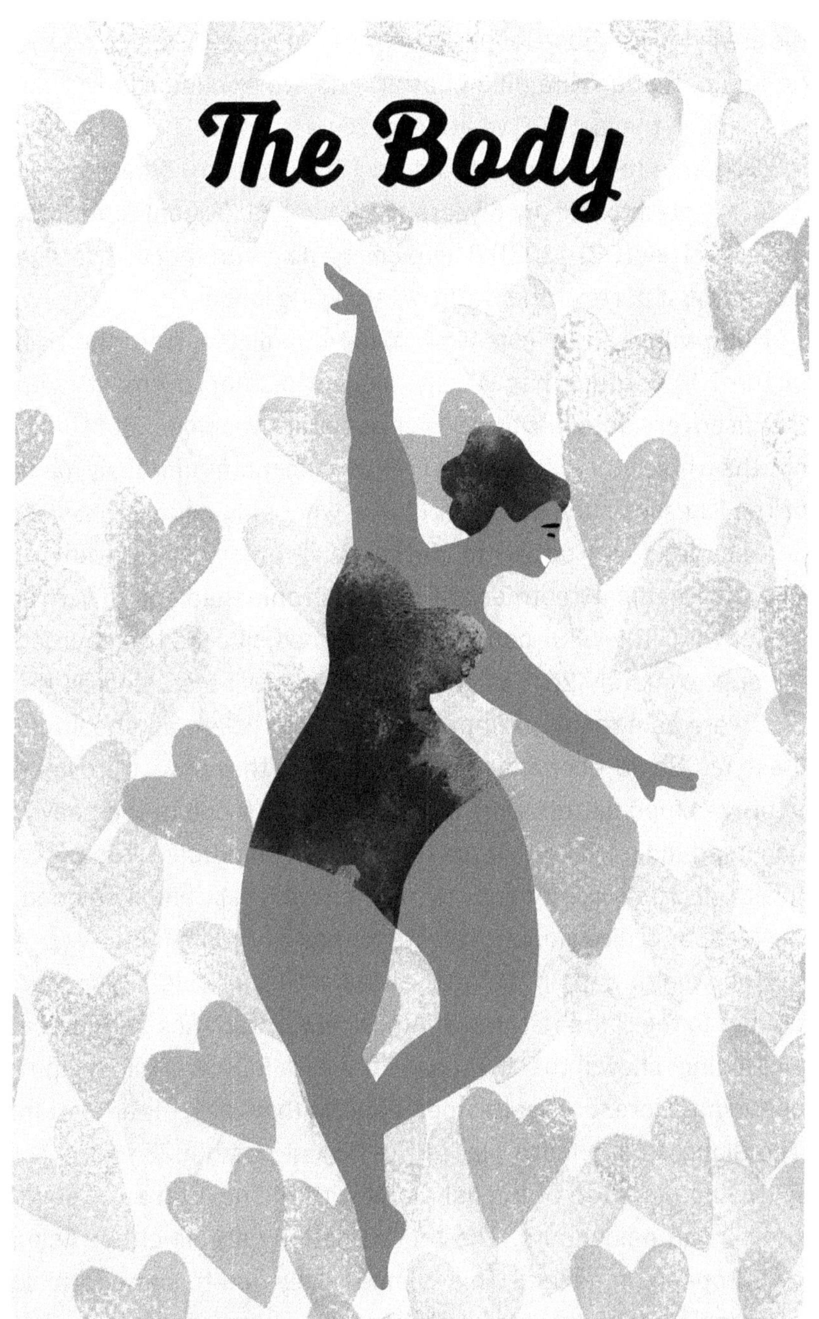
The Body

We are living for much longer, it's a fact - the body is surviving the rigours of modern life much better. The average life expectancy has risen in the last 200 years from 26 years in 1820 to 72,9 years in 2020, due to a variety of factors. (Statista.com) What's more, it is expected to rise by 5 years to 78 by 2050 (Global Burden of Disease Study (GBD) 2021). There can be no doubt that on average across most parts of the world we are living longer.

Many will say, the advent of modern medicine, from the turn of the 20th Century, has largely caused this improvement, with the discovery of penicillin and various other vaccines. But this is not the whole story, if the data is examined more rigorously many of the illnesses such as tuberculosis, whooping cough, measles, and scarlet fever began to decline well before the advent of effective medical treatments. The British epidemiologist Thomas McKeown (1912-1988) concluded that medicine had accounted for approximately 20% of the reduced death rates, and all the rest were as a result of improved sanitation, diet, and healthier lifestyles. Socio-economically, the advent of the railways provided improved food distribution, bringing fresher foods to the heavily occupied industrial cities, this also had a significant impact on health. Today it is fair to say, we have never really had it so good, despite some dire global hotspots for poverty and famine.

The wealth gap, in general, allows richer people live longer, but not in the United States of America! All statistics for medical well-being shows the USA not to be doing so well, despite spending more on health, per capita, than any other nation. The Global Health Index places the USA at number 35 on the list with Singapore top of the list along with the next three all being their Asian neighbours. The top 20 nations are all either Asian or European. In general, this is most likely due to some form of affordable healthcare, good diet and exercise compared to that of America. The bad news for South Africa, ranked at 129/167, on the same list, is that our health suffers due to poverty, high unemployment, a poor public healthcare system, and poor diet.

Our body is our only vehicle we have to journey through a relatively short life, with current limits being around the average life expectancy. The oldest person living right now in 2025 is 116. Today nothing is really made to last. In a throw-away society, we just replace something when it's broken. Although some of our body parts can be replaced relatively easily this way, such as hip joints, most of our internal organs are really very difficult to replace when diseased or cease to function, such as heart, lungs, kidneys, and liver. Of course, it's not impossible but still very costly and risky. It is much better, where we can, to take care of our one-and-only body so that it lasts as long as it can.

Our bodies are also blessed with a strong survival mechanism called resilience. This is the body's ability to adapt to challenges, maintain stamina and strength, and recover quickly and efficiently - our ability to 'bounce back' in other words. This mechanism is designed to save us for short periods, and in moments of crisis. But resilience can be abused. We can adapt to poor diets, absorb the aches and pains from poor posture, from sitting too much, and slouching on the sofa all day with no exercise. Our body will cope, but not without a cost, something is degenerating as a result of that lack of care. After a time, parts will start to ache and things go wrong. Our bodies need care and maintenance if they are to last, for a life of fulfilment.

#20

See the body as whole and complete

"Our bodies are our gardens - our wills are our gardeners."

William Shakespeare (c1564-1616)
English playwright, poet, and actor.

"Keeping your body healthy is an expression of gratitude to the whole cosmos - the trees, the clouds, everything."

Thich Nhat Hanh (1926-2022)
Vietnamese Buddhist monk, peace activist, prolific author, poet, and teacher.

"Health is a state of complete physical, mental, and social well-being and not merely the absence of disease or infirmity."

Constitution of the World Health Organization.

Did you know that most of the clinical trials of drugs on humans are designed to ensure that there is only one drug administered, and that the participant only has the one condition the drug is aiming to impact This it is said, eliminates 'confounding variables', all those things that might cloud the results. This is where we have arrived with western medicine, the piece-meal application of a treatment or drug, and an avoidance of understanding of the whole. The body is a very complex system-of-systems. We have brain surgeons, skin doctors, mouth doctors, back doctors, heart doctors - you name the body part or disease there is a specialist doctor for it. In fact, there are several hundred medical specialties and subspecialties! Their purpose is to focus predominantly on that specific element. Where is the 'whole body doctor'? That would be your GP, let's assume, whose appointments last for 15 minutes, with a script and a follow-up appointment if you do not recover. To be fair there is also an increase in the provision of holistic medicine, which does cater for the whole and not individual parts.

Just who designed this thing our soul and mind resides in for the nominal age of 70, for our life expectancy? Note also, women live decidedly longer than men, largely due to men having riskier lifestyles. Surely someone must have designed us; either God did or we evolved from a single cell in a puddle of water, you decide. One thing is for sure, we certainly have an amazing body. Humans are around 99,9% the same, in terms of shared genes, but each person is unique, that's the importance of the last 0,1%.

Although there are a few parts we can survive without, body parts such as, the appendix, gall bladder, wisdom teeth, coccyx, and male nipples. All these are termed vestigial organs or ones that have no purpose, and are a vestige, or leftover, from our ancestors and we have around 100 of them! Generally however, the body is one amazing super system, each part working in unison to some perfect rhythm we have yet to totally understand.

In your own journey to good health, and in maintaining it, what makes you take healthy whole-body choices? How you exercise, sleep, eat and drink, what you expose your body to, and what you expose your mind to, and how you interact with your greater higher power determines your health. In your wholeness you really are a divine trinity, of mind, body, and soul. Respecting this wholeness through life is certainly key to optimising your lifestyle.

Life Hack #1

Certain situations induce creativity of my mind and soul. For me one is flying and the other the gym's cross-trainer. I don't know why but the sensation of flying and the ease at which I can stand on the stationary cross-trainer and exercise, frees me up to having the biggest, big-picture creative thoughts. Proof that the body is always, and continuously whole-body working. If I don't capture the thoughts there and then, they are gone for good. Where does this happen to you? Find it and try going there more often. Your phone has a dictation app to capture your thoughts, believe me you'll need it!

Life Hack #2

Try Body Stress Release! I have to say that somewhere in the book. We really do practise a whole-body technique, and though you may go with an ache or a pain here and there, it will certainly open your eyes to a whole new self-healing body experience. We work along the complete spine, in the muscle tissue, where around 90% of the body's nerve function pass through, and it's a very gentle technique to experience. Go to www.bodystressrelease.com and you'll see a 'Find a Practitioner' button to find the nearest one. Your body will love you for trying it.

As it is, there are many parts, but one body. The eye cannot say to the hand, "I don't need you!" And the head cannot say to the feet, "I don't need you!" so that there should be no division in the body, but that its parts should have equal concern for each other. If one part suffers, every part suffers with it; if one part is honoured, every part rejoices with it.

1 Corinthians 12: 20-24

#21

Stress creates deficiencies

"The greatest weapon against stress is our ability to choose one thought over another."

William James (1842-1910)
American philosopher, psychologist, and the first educator to offer a psychology course in the United States.

"Stress is the trash of modern life - we all generate it but if you don't dispose of it properly, it will pile up and overtake your life."

Danzae Pace (Not Known)
A person.

"Stress is an ignorant state. It believes that everything is an emergency."

Natalie Goldberg (1948-present)
American popular author, and speaker. She is best known for a series of books which explore writing as a Zen practice.

"I'm so stressed out" - the most common phrase I hear from my clients at their first appointment. I reassure them, they came to the right place! They are often suffering some type of body stress or locked-in tension, which is causing them an ache or pain or some other body malady. Headaches, cramps, nerve pains, constipation, may all be attributable to stress. But not all stress is bad for you, did you know there is some good stress too?

Experts have failed to agree on a single definition of stress, it can be many things to many different people. It has therefore, been difficult to measure stress quantitatively; there are only soft or qualitative indictors to stress levels. Many people therefore, have very different ideas with respect to their definition of stress. There are three stress states covering the body where we can either be: calm (or unstressed), in a state of stress that is good or healthy (Eustress) and an unhealthy or distressed state.

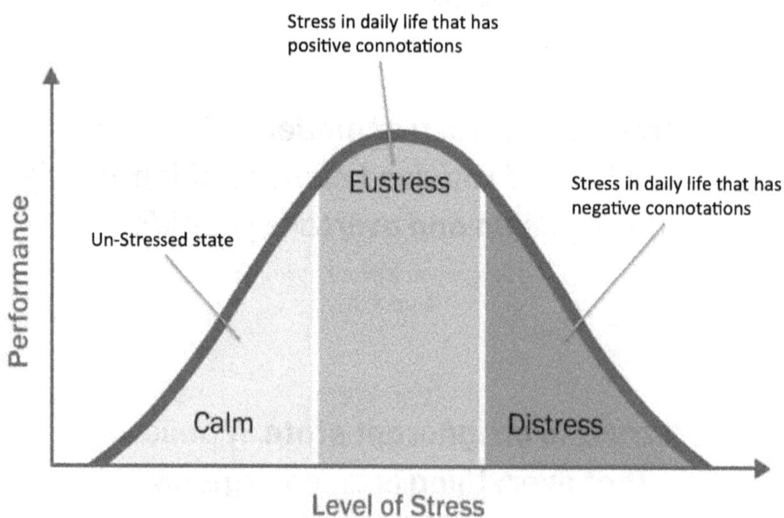

Reference: The American Institute of Stress

From a state of calmness, we may experience good stress, such as the elation or adrenalin rush from competing in a race; that first kiss, a graduation ceremony or a bungee jump. This type of stress is normal and quite healthy for the mind and body, and is developmental. Our body can also go into distress however, this is the interaction between the external environment or conditions interacting with our body's internal biochemical and physiological systems in a cognitive or thinking process.

The types of stress we may suffer from originate from; Mechanical Stress (such as bad posture and traumas to the body; Emotional Stress (things we worry about at work or home) and Chemical Stress (largely from processed food intake). It takes energy to lock-in and store stress, and that energy has to come from somewhere. Basically, stress locked into the body is an 'energy vampire', sucking the energy away from our day-to-day activities, and reducing their efficiencies. It certainly is 'the silent killer' and can result in fatigue, lethargy anxiety, depression, and heart disease, amongst many other potential ailments.

Life Hack #1

The top stress buster has to be exercise! I often hear, *"But I am busy all day running around, isn't that exercise?"* Sadly, no it is not, that is really just more bad stress. Exercise would be defined as raising your heart rate, and doing whatever activity you chose for around 45 minutes, 3 times a week or preferably more and preferably outside. The green trees and the blue sky are natural stress busters, which complement the physical dimension. If you currently do nothing - start with simple walking, something we are designed to do with little extra effort.

Do not be anxious about anything, but in every situation, by prayer and petition, with thanksgiving, present your requests to God.

Philippians 4:6

#22

Mask on first

"To love oneself is the beginning of a lifelong romance."

Oscar Wilde (1854-1900)
Irish poet and playwright famous for his sharp wit.

"It's all about falling in love with yourself and sharing that love with someone who appreciates you, rather than looking for love to compensate for a self-love deficit."

Eartha Kitt (1927-2008)
American singer and actress known for her highly distinctive singing style.

"Your self-worth is determined by you. You don't have to depend on someone telling you who you are."

Beyoncé (1981-present)
American singer, songwriter, and businesswoman.

I am sure you have heard the words *"In the unlikely event of a loss in cabin pressure, oxygen masks will drop from the overhead compartments."* When we are instructed to *"Put your own mask on first before assisting anyone else."* Pretty selfish you might think, to go 'me-first' but it makes perfect sense. Otherwise, in assisting someone else, before being safe you might become a victim AND interfere in someone else's safety. Double whammy! The principle however, is sound, you cannot help someone else if you haven't helped yourself first or put yourself in the best mental and physical shape to do so. You can best help others from a position of your own wellbeing and strength.

In my own BSR practice, I see this a great deal in parents and especially mums, sad to say. A mother's natural instinct to love and nurture, and they often do this at a cost to their own physical and mental health. I call it the 'Busy-Mum Syndrome." By putting others first, their children and their husband, pretty much all the time, the self-love batteries at some point are going to deplete to nothing. Of course, these days this is not the sole prerogative, of Mums, Dads may also suffer. No 'me-time', no time for exercise, no time for anything else apart from working hard to support the family, is never sustainable. Something will give, sooner or later, either in the body, the mind or in a relationship.

As Ewald said *"If I'm exhausted or ill, I cannot help anyone."* It's the mask-on first principle, and the basis of self-care, self-respect and self-love. Try to get out of the selfish mindset when taking time for you; you need it, others need you and, in the words of the famous make-up brand, do it - *"Because you're worth it."* And you really are worth it, view self-care as an investment, and not only for you, for others around you as well. Everyone you interact with will benefit from a strong and capable you, and you will radiate the love you've invested in yourself manyfold to those close to you. Replace the 'double whammy' with a win-win.

Life Hack #1

The greatest gift to yourself is time. Time to do something for you, that brings you joy, makes you happy and gives you something in return. A power nap or siesta, lunch with a friend, a sundowner on the beach or a walk in the park with your dog. What is it that brings you peace in a hectic day? This is your homework and yours alone, find it, know it and do it daily.

Life Hack #2

Stay hydrated, enough water in the body's system is crucial for a wide variety of reasons. Should be easy right? Yet plain ordinary water seems to be my own kryptonite. I make resolutions, buy new fancy bottles, and buy special water, yet still cannot manage to drink what I should do each day. Water is a body sustainment basic. Even mild dehydration can cause fatigue, poor concentration, and irritability, so make sure you're staying hydrated!

Don't you know that you yourselves are God's temple and that God's Spirit dwells in your midst?

1 Corinthian 3:16

#23

The need for rest

"If tonight my soul may find her peace in sleep, and sink in good oblivion, and in the morning wake like a new opened flower then I have been dipped again in God, and new created."

D.H. Lawrence (1885-1930)
English novelist, short-story writer, poet, playwright, literary critic, travel writer, essayist, and painter.

"If you get tired, learn to rest, not to quit."

Banksy (Who knows?)
English street artist, political activist, and film director whose identity remains unconfirmed and the subject of speculation.

"Real rest feels like every cell is thanking you for taking care of you. It's calm, not full of checklists and chores. It's simple: not multitasking; not fixing broken things."

Jennifer Williamson (1973-present)
American attorney, Democratic politician, and political strategist.

One of the questions I ask my clients in recording their stressful journey is *"How well do you sleep?"* It is a key indicator of how healthy they are, usually healthy people sleep about 8 hours per day. Sleeping at night in bed, accounts for one-third of our life! It is the time our body needs to recover from the busy day we have just had and to prepare us for the one to come. People who sleep well, get sick less often, maintain a healthy weight better, and it lowers their risk of serious health problems, like diabetes and heart disease. In turn, it lowers stress and helps you to think more clearly and perform better. (The Office of Disease Prevention and Health Promotion, USA). The benefits for a normal healthy body are obvious, but much more important when we are sick. *"For healing to take place, body needs to rest."* This was Ewald's maxim on rest, and advice to his clients. Sadly, many of those with illnesses refuse the take this onboard as a part of a credible healing strategy. There are seven types of rest; physical, mental, emotional, sensory, creative, social, and spiritual. Each type focuses on a different aspect of our lives and at some point, each element needs to be rested and undertake a period of refreshment.

Healing also requires a change to our health status, from unhealthy to healthy (or a reversion to normal healthy state). Part of the brain, the amygdala, interprets change as a threat and releases the hormones for fear, fight or flight. Your body is actually protecting you from change. That is why so many people in an organisation, when presented with a new initiative or idea - even a good one, with plenty of benefits, will resist it. It is the same on a healing journey, many become comfortable and complacent in their illness and unconsciously resist the potential for healing changes, especially new ones. Unfortunately, some still believe that rest looks like laziness to others around them.

Another way to rest is the 'power nap' during the day, say for around 20 minutes. This might be to counter the sleep debt from the poor night's sleep or just because you need it! It's the Mediterranean principle of the *siesta*. Go to Spain on holiday and almost everything shuts down from 2-4 pm daily, as it's pretty hot and it also promotes productivity during the rest of the day. In 29 years in the Army, you learn to sleep anywhere and anytime you can, all the time. Sleep and rest is viewed as key ingredient towards high performance in the most difficult of situations. Take rest when your body is telling you it needs it, do not resist, it really is counter intuitive.

Life Hack #1

We have two nervous systems and at the basic level we can fuel, either the 'rest and digest' one or the 'fight and flight' one - not both at the same time. Guess what? - lunch on the move isn't going to work, you won't rest, and you won't digest you food correctly. Best to have a lunch break! Daily! It pays back and supports physical and mental health and reduces stress levels - ready for the afternoon session. You should then be rested and have a more productive afternoon and arrive home not overly tired.

Life Hack #2

Take a break - even if you don't think you need one. It may be another daily one. Even if you really did have a lunch break. Now tea-at-three time, have a cuppa and relax, its only 15 minutes maximum. Or the break maybe for a long weekend, now and then or that holiday you've been putting off for months? Book it, and go. No doubt your body really needs it, and will appreciate it, and will pay you back the dividend!

Life Hack #3

Do a 'Sleep Audit'. Sleep is the best form of rest and its length and quality need to be effective to provide your body with the most return on the sleep investment. If we are talking hours then the Mayo Clinic recommends more than 7 hours per night, and continuously, not broken, for the average adult. But by reviewing your sleep quality and how you feel when you wake up you'll know if it's good enough. If not, time to go my web page www.simonbsr.co.za/ and look under the resources tab, where you'll find 'How to Counter Stress' - where I give 9 Top Tips for a good night's sleep.

My soul finds rest in God alone; my salvation comes from him. He alone is my rock and my salvation; he is my fortress, I will never be shaken.

Psalm 62:1

#24

The body doesn't know how to lie

"The body never lies."

Martha Graham (1894-1991)
American modern dancer and choreographer, whose style, the Graham technique, reshaped American dance.

"The body tells the truth regardless of if we speak its language or not... Often my practice has focused on trying to meet my body where it is, instead of constantly trying to get it to meet me where I am."

Lama Rod Owens (Not Known)
American lama in the Kagyu School of Tibetan Buddhism.

"From the moment you're born to the moment you die, the only thing you can rely on is the sensation of being in your body."

www.yourtango.com/

Imagine your body as your own special vehicle through life, and it takes you from 0 to 70 in, well, 70 years! Your body has a lifespan for sure, but we never know for how long. Our body and our traditional five senses is how we experience the outside world, and how we interact with each other. The body, as we have read, is guided by our three minds or intelligences, the brain, the heart, and the gut (for intuition), and contains that fuzzy part we're coming to, our soul or our inner-being.

There are other types of memory or intelligence at work too, such as muscle memory. We can create this to train our body for sport for example. Also, there is somatic memory, this is the idea that the body stores stress and trauma in the body structure, and not just the mind. This part we often see in the release of locked-in tension in our Body Stress Release practices. Then there is cellular memory; the idea that non-brain cells have memories. An example is those who have organ transplants, they often have 'memories' of their donors, even though this is considered impossible. Cells do however, have a memory, else we would not survive. Cells can remember damage and repair responses, and research shows that gene codes can be affected by physical traumas. These may also be passed down genetically through generations, otherwise known as generational trauma. One of the first papers to note the presence of intergenerational trauma appeared in 1966, when, South African born Canadian psychiatrist Vivian Rakoff, MD, and colleagues documented high rates of psychological distress among children of Holocaust survivors.

These are the ways in which the body is remembering life and body experiences and telling you the truth, and your own truth, unique to your own journey. Although we all have roughly the same skills and abilities, we all bring them into being in very different ways. Even the preprogrammed responses such as 'fight or flight' are all initiated to your own body truth. Thus, the body never lies, its only our logical mind, or deceitful emotional heart that can create the lies from 'alternative facts'. This was a euphemism created by the Trump Administration to legitimise lies or falsehoods. In our bodies we do this all the time, it tells the truth, we make it into a falsehood. Men get testicular cancer, which is curable if caught early, it starts with a small but truthful undeniable lump usually to which the brain rationalises *"it is my vasectomy scar"* or *"I'm sure it's always been there."* Men do this a lot! Men especially so, need to undertake their health checks more often.

Life Hack #1

Do a full body scan, and no, not an MRI. This one you can do at home, any time. Have you ever replied to someone "I'm fine" when they ask after your well-being, when in truth you are not fine, not fine at all. Sit down and have a conversation with your body, mentally ask it *"How are you today?"* Step 1 is to listen - Step 2, is to really hear the answer - Step 3, is to write it down. Do a 'full service', just like the Discovery Insurance Multipoint Check they do on your car. Start at the feet and end at the head. No need to make a list - your brain is intimately connected to your body, it is managing it every second of every day. Take a print-out and see what the report says. Time for a doctor's check-up or a screening event? Book it today, the results of them also never lie.

"The heart is deceitful above all things and desperately sick; who can understand it?"

Jeremiah 17:9

#25

Listen to your body

"If you listen to your body when it whispers, you won't have to listen when it screams."

Anon.

"Your body is speaking to you. It always speaks to you."

Renée Fishman (Not Known)
American creative spirit, intellectual, student of life, and specialist in holistic help.

"It's all about tuning out the noise, tuning out all the stuff that simply doesn't move the game forward - the doubt, the personal agendas, the often deafening fear of judgment and the need to please - so that you can ultimately get to that place of quiet, of calm, where you can focus on what really matters."

Bonnie Hammer (1950-present)
American network and studio executive.

From early in our lives, we learn to ignore our body and how it communicates with us. We're conditioned to numb physical sensations with pain killers, ignore messages of exhaustion, and pay no credence to the whispers and warnings, that our bodies signal to us of pending illness or disease. We are beings made to cope, adjust, manage out the issues, to do all those safety-critical things we do so well every day; driving, cooking, looking after the kids, the list is endless. Our body can be its own worst enemy unless we learn to understand and listen to it regularly.

Your body carries profound intelligence, programmed into your DNA, and far deeper than the conscious mind can ever hope to know. It speaks to you in dozens of ways. The problem is that we don't know how to listen anymore, we've lost touch, as we've moved further away from nature, with its rhythms and cycles. If you truly listen, it will tell you with whom to spend more time, and from whom to stay away, when to rest, when to push harder, when to be active, and when to be calm. It will even tell you what work is most aligned for you and where to focus your efforts. But you have to listen to it, hear it and understand the response required. Then take some action to fix it. Pain, aching, stiffness, lethargy, and tiredness are some of the key things to watch out for, but so are cramps, repetitive infection or illness, changes in body temperature, all these can be indicators something is wrong - some type of body stress or issue.

The ability to listen to your inner quiet messages about what will heal you is called listening to your 'whispers'! There is so much noise and distraction in the world - not to mention whatever fears, baggage and anxieties might get in our way. Learning to hear those whispers is key to understanding your health journey.

Body stress may result in:

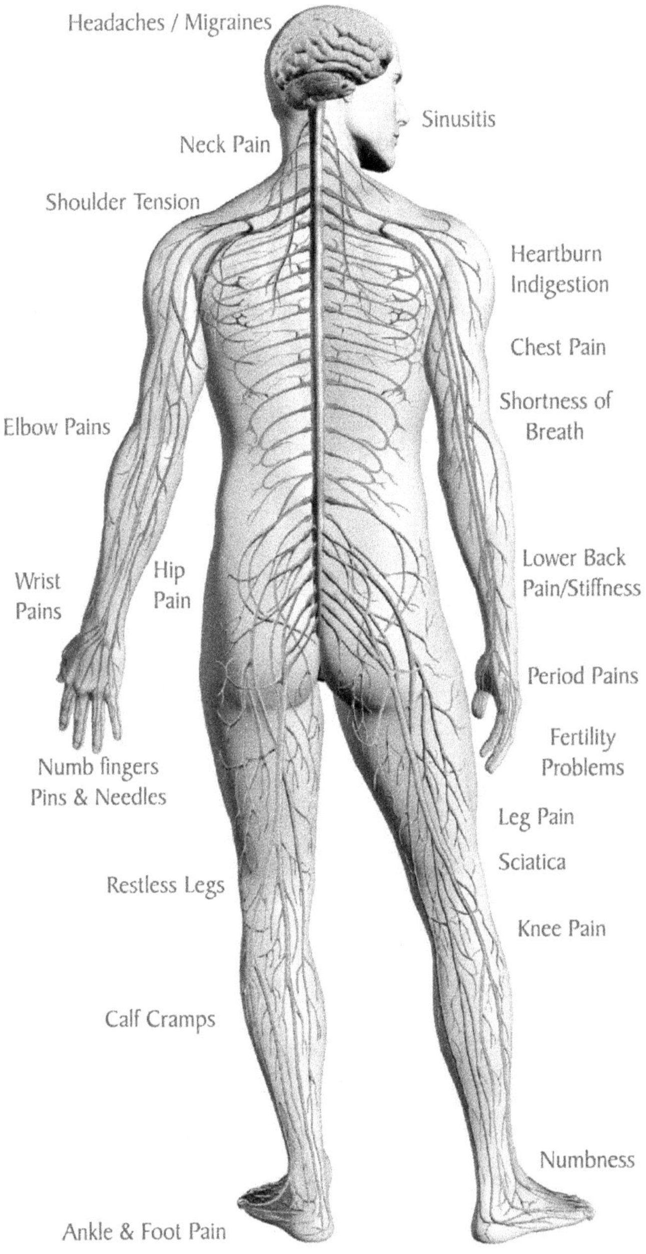

Life Hack #1

Get grounded - by a reconnection to the Earth and the stillness nature can bring to your body. It is a way to reconnect with the inner you and tune out life's noise. It is also simple - take off your shoes AND socks and go walk outside on the grass, soil or a lovely sandy beach for at least ten to twenty minutes a day. Scientifically you're actually earthing your body to the natural electric charge of the earth and allowing it to return to a neutral level by creating a conductivity between the charged-up you and earth beneath your feet. Try to do this daily. This also links to creating a resonance to the Earth which we will read about later.

The eye is the lamp of the body. If your eyes are healthy, your whole body will be full of light. But if your eyes are unhealthy, your whole body will be full of darkness. If then the light within you is darkness, how great is that darkness!

Matthew 6:22-23

#26

Body makes the best of a bad situation

"As long as you are breathing, there is more right with you than there is wrong, no matter how ill or how hopeless you may feel."

Jon Kabat-Zinn (1944-present)
American professor emeritus of medicine, and the creator of the Stress Reduction Clinic, and the Center for Mindfulness in Medicine.

"You may encounter many defeats, but you must not be defeated. In fact, it may be necessary to encounter the defeats so you can know who you are, what you can rise from, how you can still come out of it."

Maya Angelou (1928-2014)
American memoirist, poet, and civil rights activist.

"The only easy day was yesterday."

Mark Bissonnette (1976-present)
American former US Navy SEAL.

The body has an in-built capability to adapt and survive. That's why we have managed to make it to the top of the food chain as a species. We have an in-built survival mechanism and an innate ability to adapt and survive, both as a race and as human beings. Our coping mechanism vary as individuals, but we come designed and pre-loaded to survive! One person's bad day is another's easy day. From having a bad headache to being shipwrecked on a desert island, we can draw on resources our conscious mind has no concept of. We literally have no idea what we can endure and survive, at all levels of our existence from the cell level to our higher spiritual consciousness.

Mark Bissonnette's quote came from his autobiographical account of service as a US Navy SEAL, called *No Easy Day,* and sums up that once the hardest of hard days is over, the next day, is really the hardest to overcome. The body works daily to adapt and survive. One of our survival mechanisms is the RAS or the Reticular Activating System (RAS). Defined as, *"a bundle of nerves that sits in your brainstem, its job is to regulate behavioural arousal, consciousness and motivation. The RAS is able to control what incoming information you're aware of, so that you'll be motivated to behave in a certain way."* (www.lifeexchangesolutions.com/) It sits there functioning like a guard and filters out what information you really don't need and allows through what you do need at that instant. We just cannot cope with every piece of sensory information. Even our phenomenal brain power cannot process it all. We live our lives on a partial representation of ourselves and of our environment.

Two examples of how this works - you see a tiger running towards you for the first time, the brain processes right now to do something, and quickly. The second is driving your car; ever driven somewhere on 'automatic pilot', you were still in control, but it was like the car was driving itself. In the first instance the RAS lets through the signals and in the second example it is active only to use what it really, really needs for the activity of driving. We tend to do the same with pain signals, those which are vital to the healing process. If they persist for long periods of time the RAS, tells the body, *"Filter them out - we can cope"* - and guess what we do - make the best of a bad situation. Often, we do this for stress-related events and with longer-term, locked-in tension. I see this in my BSR practice almost daily.

Life Hack #1

Dial in your goals! There is a suggestion that you can train your RAS, by linking your subconscious thoughts to your conscious ones. It is another way of setting your intent. A daily focus on your goals will 'reset' the RAS and allow that information through which is always important to those goals. It will reveal the people, opportunities, and information required to achieve them and NOT filter them out.

Life Hack #2

Why not make the best out of a better situation, and not a bad one. Doesn't that sound amazing? What is your body's current 'bad situation?' What are you coping with and what signals are you filtering out? You just don't know. You did the full body scan, but now let's do something different, here you need to tap into the RAS and find what was filtered out. The memory is there somewhere, and it's recent. What tiny, niggly sensation did you filter out or ignore? Tap into it and magnify it, see what your gut is telling you to do, time for some body-review or fixing remedy... you'll know it once you find it!

Do not be anxious about anything, but in every situation, by prayer and petition, with thanksgiving, present your requests to God.

Philippians 4:6

#27

Exercise with wisdom, think with clarity

"Movement is a medicine for creating change in a person's physical, emotional, and mental states."

Carol Welch-Baril (Not known)
Neuromuscular therapist and somatic instructor
who coined the slogan for the Movement Therapy sector.

"If you don't make time for exercise, you'll probably have to make time for illness."

Robin Sharma (1964-present)
Canadian writer, best known for his book series,
The Monk Who Sold His Ferrari.

"Physical fitness is not only one of the most important keys to a healthy body, it is the basis of dynamic and creative intellectual activity."

John F Kennedy (1917-1963)
Kennedy, often referred to as JFK, was the 35th president of the United States,
serving from 1961 until his assassination in 1963.

"Exercise with wisdom, think with clarity", this would be a reasonable summary of my 29 years in the military. There were plenty of days with bad situations, many physical, some mental and some moral dilemmas to overcome, but being fit for purpose was always important to getting through each day. With all the sayings and wisdoms I have seen from Ewald this is the only one that relates to exercise and being fit. We have already been through an exercising of the mind, now it's the body's turn, and for us to think about how we get fit and maintain that fitness.

If you're already not sure what 'exercise' means, here is a reasonable definition, *"at least 150 minutes of moderate aerobic activity. Or get at least 75 minutes of vigorous aerobic activity a week. You can also get an equal mix of the two types. The aim is to exercise most days of the week."* (The Mayo Clinic). Easy enough for most of us to achieve, you would imagine? However, we all lead busy lives, and often for many exercise can just wait. Because - yes, you've got it... 'the body makes the best of a bad situation.' In this case it can manage without exercise for sure, but over a period will start to degenerate. It is often stated; 'Sitting is the new smoking' meaning too much inactivity can be a definite hazard to healthy well-being.

The analogy I use with my clients are their quite shiny cars! Each comes with maintenance plan to keep it smooth and running in peak condition. Why? - well these costly machines that move us from A to B are really worth looking after. Sadly, they're NOT an investment but are worth keeping in a great condition to be reliable. Research shows, that in a lifetime, we might own eight or more cars. I hope you see where I'm going...

Your life expectancy is around 70-80 years depending on your particular demographic, and guess what? you only get one bio-mechanical machine to move you around from A to B. How much are you spending to maintain yours? Or are you using the South African taxi driver mentality - to fix it only when the wheel drops off. The western medicine model is very much considered to be 'fix me when I'm broken', but the health and wellness sector is now moving towards a 'keep me healthy to avoid illness' model. Here is the thinking with clarity part - think more like a human body owner and less like a car owner. Start your own routine and thorough maintenance plan today.

Life Hack #1

Let me start with the non-exerciser, or those struggling in some way to find something to do. Walk, walk, and walk some more. We are really very well designed for this purpose. It is a natural activity and we do it every day, but often not enough. Start with a little and often, the end of the street, every other day, then daily, then the following week around the block and build up to say, an hour three times a week as a fair target. That would be about 3% of your waking time in a week, 3 hours for a minimum is not too much to ask for, is it?

Life Hack #2

Keep moving even when you're not supposed to! What does this mean? If 'sitting really is the new smoking', why are you sitting so much? We lead an increasingly sedentary life-style in front of the computer screen, driving, watching TV, for easily more than 8 hours a day. Try a better process for kick-starting all those bodily systems that get sluggish while sitting; get up from the PC every 20 minutes, take cell phone calls while walking, take lunchtime walks. Find small ways to add in more daily movement. All these rather than being time wasters will actually increase productivity!

For physical training is of some value, but godliness has value for all things, holding promise for both the present life and the life to come.

1 Timothy 4:8

#28

The body's wisdom is more powerful than the mind

"Wisdom is not a product of schooling but of the lifelong attempt to acquire it."

Albert Einstein (1879-1955)
German-born theoretical physicist who is best known for the theories of relativity.

"Intelligence is present everywhere in our bodies... our own inner intelligence is far superior to any we can try to substitute from the outside."

Deepak Chopra (1946-present)
Indian American author, new age guru, and alternative-medicine advocate.

"If you're willing to pay attention to and dialogue with what's happening inside of you, you'll find that your body already knows the answers about how to live a full, present, connected, and healthy life."

Hillary L McBride (Not known)
A Canadian-registered psychologist, and award-winning researcher, and the former host of the Other People's Problems, and the Holy/Hurt podcasts.

These days we are bombarded with information, disinformation, misinformation, conspiracy theories, and marketing campaigns designed to capture our attention and our minds. Often this is in pursuit of something we are told we need to make us, healthy, better, fitter, stronger or wiser! The competition for our minds and spending power in relation to our mind, body, and soul is fierce, and led by a plethora of 'experts'. Meanwhile our body, with thousands of years' worth of experience in survival, has been developing and acquiring knowledge and wisdom.

Did you know our bodies are self-healing? We cut ourselves, we bleed, we scab, we scar, and heal and recover. This is an obvious event for physical wounds we take for granted, and what's best is, we do nothing, we're programmed to do this. It is the same for many of the aspects of our body's development and growth. If we do the basics well, then our body functions pretty well too. Eat a variety of healthy foods, drink enough clean water, breathe clean air, and exercise regularly then our bodies stand the best chance of serving us well and continue to self-regulate and self-heal.

The 'logical mind' is often our worst enemy in this regard. Powerful and clever, but vulnerable to outside intelligence, telling us its quicker or easier - this way or that way. Learning to trust our own bodies in a world increasingly filled full of fear and doubt is often a difficult concept. The vaccines and cancer debates are two examples for which I would never profess or feel remotely experienced, let alone qualified to recommend answers on. Your world view and wisdom will have to prevail. When faced with debates like this, I usually start with motivation. What's someone's motivation for a view that might be contrary to what my body and its experience is telling me, then take it from there.

Finally, the mind creates its own 'reality'. Already over stimulated with sensory inputs and now overwhelmed with choices of every kind in a complex world, the mind creates a simple version it can cope with. We often have to rationalise a complex dataset from many sources into a version we can cope with, including all the information regarding what to do with our body. Our body, on the other hand, has all the wisdom and processing capability you can ever imagine to be healthy. All you must do is supply it with the correct nutrition, keep it moving, don't abuse it in any way, and allow it rest when it needs it. It's so simple, yet we often get it so very wrong.

Life Hack #1

There is no life hack other than - do the work daily to be healthy and respect and listen to your body's wisdom. No short-cuts with this one! Be wise in your daily choices, and listen to your body's gut wisdom, it is usually correct. You know what you can do more of and what you need to cut out. Make these two lists and start with that simple hack today.

Is not wisdom found among the aged?
Does not long life bring understanding?

Job12:12

#29

The body is a natural "detoxer"

"Detoxing gives your body a break and allows its self-cleansing and self-healing processes to kick in."

Anon.

"We live in a toxic environment that is damaging our bodies and minds."

Doctor Mark Hyman (1959-present)
American physician and author.

"Detoxification is a means of reconnecting with your body, mind, and spirit."

Anon.

Detoxification (or detox for short) is, *"a process or period of time in which one abstains from, or rids the body of toxic, or unhealthy substances."* (Oxford English Dictionary). In other words, a cleaning or cleansing process. One of the most important features of the body is that it eliminates things it doesn't need, can't use or that can harm it. The body has its own filter systems for this, consisting mainly of the kidneys and liver for everything ingested. In an emergency, the body eliminates other toxic ingestions as vomit or diarrhoea. Our bodies are generally very good at this process and need little else in doing the job.

That said, we live in an increasingly toxic and chemical infused world! Our tinned, packaged, and processed food chain is heavily chemicalised, with food containing colourants, flavourings, stabilisers and all manner of industrialised ingredients. The water can contain, Anti Retro Viral (ARVs), contraceptives, and micro-plastics, and the air and chemical fragrances we breath in can contain any type and level of toxic load. Similarly, any products applied to the outside of our bodies, from skin creams, powders, and cleansing products can all be absorbed into our bloodstream, this time with the added danger of no filtration or any ability to eliminate anything toxic.

Despite the body having a natural ability to detoxify, it is currently being saturated with chemicals from every source and direction. This prompted the growth, of industries seeking your 'detox-$$$'. For 2023, the global detox products market stands at an annual figure of US$ 56,13 billion and predicting an annual growth of about 5%. This however, is not a new industry; the health conscious Egyptians and Romans all famously had spas and detoxification practices 2 000 years ago. So, do they work?

Again research suggests that most detoxification processes have limited benefits and what benefits they do have are usually sort-term fixes for longer-term issues. This does not include drug rehabilitation, which is entirely different with about a 68% success rate. Usually it's best to rest, cut out as many chemicals as possible, and drink plenty of water. In many of the spa treatments etc, the 'feel-good factor', is also at play and, although some detox treatments may not be totally needed, they can feel good and generally enhance our overall mental well-being, while not always benefitting a detoxification process.

Life Hack #1

Read food labels and packets and product packages. Just trying to read the names of some of the chemicals will be hard enough! Then ask yourself - what exactly is that? - 'Mr. Google' will help you better understand what is going into your body. Switching your body to a healthier diet will more actively promote the body's natural ability to detox than any other external process. But if you want a moment's joy, book the spa as well!

Life Hack #2

Your body can already detox - but prevention is better than cure, follow these tips to maintain a healthy detoxified body which can do it all for you:

- Limit alcohol intake.
- Focus on sleep - 8 hours!
- Drink more water - about 1 to 2 litres.
- Reduce your intake of sugar, salt, and processed foods.
- Eat antioxidant rich foods - pulses, berries, fruit, green leaf veggies.

- Eat foods high in probiotics, (organic is better) - garlic, onions, bananas, and oats.
- Stay active and exercise - see Wisdom #27.

You are already clean because of the word I have spoken to you.

John 15:3

#30

Daily re-energising

"The energy of the mind is the essence of life."

Aristotle (384-322BC)
Ancient Greek philosopher, and polymath.

"Passion is energy. Feel the power that comes from focusing on what excites you."

Oprah Winfrey (1954-present)
American talk show host, television producer, actress, author, and media proprietor.

"Nothing is more powerful than a person with a fully charged energy."

Paulo Coelho (1947-present)
Brazilian lyricist and novelist, his 1988 novel *The Alchemist* was an international best-seller.

The man in the Apple Store said, *"Do you mind if I check your phone's battery?"* No, I didn't mind at all - *"Ahh"* he said *"You've had the phone 1 year and it is still good at 85%."* Meaning my battery when full - only stored 85% of what it could when I bought it. Which, accounting for some shelf life etc., might have been about 95% of the full capacity at the time I bought it. Similarly, our bodies are really batteries to charge with food energy, store it in some shape or form in our metabolism and then discharge it as we do stuff, i.e., work! Even resting of course, we need some energy just to maintain a steady state.

The best way to re-energise is to rest, and then eat and drink correctly. The average adult body has an energy requirement; called the resting energy or basal need, it is around 1 200 calories/24hrs. Using an on-line calculator and the Harris-Benedict equation, the daily average intake I need, based on my age, gender, height, and weight needs to be about 2 332 calories. There are also a few other factors which play into the equation, such as ethnicity, diet, activity level, and muscle mass. Diet and what you eat is a whole library of books and advice in itself, but you need to know your body and fuel it regularly, and fuel before the hunger and thirst signs appear, otherwise you could be too late, and you will go into an energy dip.

There is no right or wrong way to physically re-energise, whether it is 7 snacks a day or 18 hours intermittent fasting, breakfast or no-breakfast regime: learn what works best for you. This may also change throughout your life too. Daily food and water intake can also change in relation to what task or activity you are doing. If you're going for a long run in preparation for the Comrade's Marathon, you're going to need to fuel more. Learning to re-energise with breaks, rests or even daily siestas, it is all part of the re-energising process, and balancing energy levels. The mind also needs a rest, think of it as a muscle. Remember how using it in your 3-hour school exams made you exhausted, the same principle applies, you must re-energise your mind daily as well.

Life Hack #1

Plan your daily food intake, at least a little, leaving things to chance can lead to bad habits. Make time for breakfast if it's your thing, pack a lunch box, keep some healthy energy bars in the car just in case. Basically, know where your next healthy intake of food is coming from, and make it a protein-based diet too - the energy delivered to your body in this form lasts longer and there is no sugar dip, after consuming carbs when the 'sugar-burn' is over.

Life Hack #2

Rest is re-energising naturally, so a full working day, including travel times, which is also work and stress, is around 10 hours per day. You will need breaks, working continuously just won't deliver the productivity you need to sustain. See also Wisdom #23 - The need for rest.

So whether you eat or drink or whatever you do, do it all for the glory of God.

1 Corinthians 10:31

#31

Love from the heart

"If I had a flower for every time I thought of you... I could walk through my garden forever."

Alfred Tennyson (1809-1892)
English poet and the Poet Laureate
during much of Queen Victoria's reign.

"Love understands love; it needs no talk."

Frances Havergal (1836-1879)
English religious poet and hymnwriter.

"To be fully seen by somebody and then be loved anyhow - this is a human offering that can border on miraculous."

Elizabeth Gilbert (1969-present)
American journalist and author, best known for her
2006 memoire *Eat, Pray, Love.*

Thankfully, love is one of those feelings in life that has no bounds or limits. Whether a mother has one child or 10 children, they are all loved the same, with no dilution along the way. Parental love is special, but then so is that for your siblings, and that for your spouse or partner, all completely special, and different from each other. I was an only child, I never felt sibling love, so I do not really appreciate or understand it, but I see how special it is to my wife who had 6 siblings when growing up. That bond and love twins have for each other must surely be 'next level' love, having shared their mother's womb together.

Love is an emotion. We feel love or feel being in love, and it is unique for everyone. It can be felt in different ways, like in the family relationships I've already described. The feeling also can be expressed in many ways, through acts of kindness or selflessness, but generally love cannot be measured in any objective way, although the body does give away subtle signs, such as pupil dilation, increased heart rate, and increased brain activity.

There is also the 'chemistry of attraction' that goes with love. Of all the emotions fuelled by hormones the biological compounds that send the love signals to the brain, did you know these bypass the logical part! Oh dear indeed, these horny little signals go straight to the amygdala, the emotional part of the brain. No wonder they cause physical sensations like butterflies in the stomach and tingling in the spine. This is love in its aroused attractive state, but the love signals we have for each other brother-to-sister, and friend-to-friend work in the same way, unfiltered and unprocessed by the logical brain. That's why the heartfelt emotions are so powerful and all consuming, and need to be guarded, kept pure, and off-set by some logic now and then and our other gut-feelings.

Life Hack #1

For living from the heart, the word kindness often springs to mind. While you might not want to love all your work colleagues, you might choose to be kind to them. Treating others as you might want them to treat you perhaps, by acceptance, love, forgiveness and kindness. Spend the day, just thinking about others and their needs, how might they need you to help them, and what is your part to them living a better life.

Life Hack #2

Whom do you need to thank? If you've been practising the living-in-gratitude hack (Wisdom #9 Life Hack #1) then sure there must be someone on those daily lists you just need to say *"Thanks, I really appreciate you for what you've been doing."* Even your partner could do with that too now and again, or Mum and Dad; Grandma and Grandad; those we love and often take for granted could do with a thank you, some heartfelt love and a little time. Guess what? It's really good for you too!

Love is patient and love is kind; love does not envy or boast; it is not arrogant or rude. it does not insist on its own way; it is not irritable or resentful; it does not rejoice at wrongdoing, but rejoices with the truth.

1 Corinthians 13:4-6

#32

The body loves gentleness

"Nothing is so strong as gentleness, nothing so gentle as real strength."

Saint Francis de Sales (1567-1622)
Francis de Sales,
Catholic prelate who served as Bishop of Geneva.

"Nature gives to every time and season some beauties of its own; and from morning to night, as from the cradle to the grave, it is but a succession of changes so gentle and easy that we can scarcely mark their progress"

Charles Dickens (1812-1870)
English novelist, journalist, short story writer and social critic.

"In a gentle way, you can shake the world."

Mahatma Ghandi (1869-1948)
Indian lawyer, anti-colonial nationalist, prime minister, and political ethicist.

It is hard to imagine that this robust body, which takes all sorts of mental and emotional stress really loves gentleness, but it really does. Of the wisdom that Ewald spoke this was probably the one most dear to his heart and had the most impact on his life. After a long journey of pain and several harsh 'clapping and slapping' modalities, it was the gentle but precise touch of his wife Gail and the technique of BSR that really started his healing journey. It was Gail's gut instinct that told her *"Here lies the truth"* after she first attended the Van Rumpt seminar which showed her how gentleness could be so powerful to helping the healing process.

BSR is a very gentle technique and acts to work with the body to release locked-in tension. Most clients are extremely surprised how gentle it is and often equally surprised by the impact and how their bodies start to release tension. I liken it to picking the most sensitive of locks, one tumbler at a time. Through an understanding of the body and using precision and feedback from 'stress-testing', a practitioner is able to provide a light impulse to prompt the body into releasing muscle tension. The technique facilitates what the body should be doing all the time, and that is self-healing. Locked-in tension from body stress is merely a barrier to the body healing itself. The Reticular Activating System (RAS) has just filtered out the pain or signals required to activate self-healing.

In other areas of our life too, changes to our bodies are best effected by small subtle changes over time. 'Life-style changes' is the buzzword these days, but the truth is that the body reacts well to small, but regular, long-term changes and they have the best chance of making a lasting impact. In exercise this is certainly true, small increments in weights produce lasting muscle changes, as do diet changes rather than 6-week crash programmes. The same is also true in learning and absorbing information for exams, better to learn daily, rather than cramming the night before. It seems we are programmed to be this way, but gentleness and subtleness are what we react best to for lasting changes and improvements to take place.

In all these changes, there is one crucial factor we need to employ in being gentle with our bodies and that is patience. No-one ever has enough time these days, and the pressure is on to save it, which is odd as you can't store it! Time relentlessly marches on and there are growing markets for crash courses, and short cuts to save time and improve. Unfortunately, the body hates short cuts, it is like we have an internal watch spring to run on its own slow time, forever resisting the pressure to change quicker than it wants to. So, be patient and steadfast in the changes you adopt with your body and mind. Measuring daily change is counter intuitive to this and it is always best to measure 'front-to-back', from where you started to where you are today. I do this often with my client's BSR session plan on their healing journey. If I ask them to measure change between sessions, they often struggle to articulate any change or improvement made. But, if I ask them about their progress since they started with me, invariably they say, *"Oh I am much better now!"*

Life Hack #1

The first hack has to be fitness and exercise as we're in the body zone! Make a plan for whatever exercise rocks your boat. Be it walking, running, cycling, swimming, hiking or something else. Set yourself a target - something you've either never done before or not done for years, and make a 6-month plan to achieve it. Over

6 to 8 weeks you should see health benefits and over 3 to 4 months you will have overhauled your lifestyle and have something new and beneficial to keep you fit and active.

Life Hack #2

Next hack is diet. There is something in your diet that's not good for you. You know it, everyone knows and yet you still eat or drink it. For me its sugar, not healthy, not wise, but still cannot stop putting it in my tea or coffee. I've always had a sweet tooth. To be fair I've come down from two good heaps of sugar to a flat one or a half a teaspoon on a good day. Maybe it's time to count the grains to reduce further, but you get my drift. Gradually reduce and reduce until you hardly notice it's there, then stop and the gentle, subtle way your body loves you, will accept the change as already done!

You have given me the shield of your salvation, and your right hand supported me, and your gentleness made me great.

Psalm 18:35

#33

Everything in its time

"Everything happens in its own time, place and pace. You may wish for something to happen. Or you may wish against its happening. But you cannot force the outcome."

Avis Viswanathan (1967-Present)
A life coach, a speaker, a happiness curator, author, and organisational transformation consultant.

"I learned that we can do anything, but we can't do everything... at least not at the same time. So think of your priorities not in terms of what activities you do, but when you do them. Timing is everything."

Dan Millman (1946-present)
American author and lecturer in the personal development field, best known for the movie Peaceful Warrior.

Time is the progression of one event over another from one that has occurred in the past, to those that are about to happen in the future. To date, time only moves in one direction, it is only possible for humans to move forwards in time and not backwards. Einstein's Theory of Relativity determined that time is relative, meaning the rate at which it passes is determined by your frame of reference. It is a human memory concept that allows time to pass quickly or to slowly drag by, depending on what we are doing. A workday can take 'forever', while a lovely two week holiday, passes 'in an instant'.

"Everything in its time" also means you can't do some things at the same time or you can't do different things at the same time. For example, you can't plant a seed and harvest at the time. There is a season which is appropriate to plant a seed and a season to harvest it. No two things like this can happen at the same time. Everything has got its own time, nature is hard-wired to grow and die and refresh, and living beings are given the same system in a circle of life. Although as living beings, we humans exist to live individual lives, we are part of a larger system called the human race.

I hope from reading so far, that you've grasped the value of time and how worthless seconds, valuable minutes, and gold-encrusted hours hold an ever-increasing worth. Although we know to be patient, and that generally, but not always, wisdom is gained in years of experience, each fleeting moment along the way should be valued and savoured. Living in mindfulness and being totally present in the moment, when you need to be, can turn the lower-value minutes and seconds into rich treasures. Let me give you an example.

I've spent very many hours sitting in a bird hide trying my best to photograph Kingfishers, and especially the Malachite Kingfisher.

It is South Africa's smallest kingfisher at around 12 centimetres, so very small and very fast. I was trying to catch it diving and catching fish. I tried believe me, but my equipment and skills were just not up to it. In the end, I did get one or two lovely shots of the bird sitting still, but to enjoy the split second it left the branch, and dived into the water returning with a fish, I just had to sit back and savour for myself. There are some things we cannot capture on a camera let alone a cell phone; they are too fleeting. Though long-term gains from patience are valuable, so are the tiny fleeting moments we experience. These you only capture in your mind. The diving kingfisher; that fleeting look someone gave you when you fell in love, the experience when someone dies in front of you - all these tiny moments, fractions of life, are too precious to miss, and add to our overall experience. Don't underestimate their power, they also happen 'in their time.'

With clients on a BSR healing journey, they often ask, *"but how long will it take? - how many sessions do I need?"* The answer for an individual on their unique healing journey is one you might expect, *"how long is a piece of string?"* Ewald would always encourage his students to never give up on clients on their path to better health saying, *"After 7 years miracles can still happen."* Everything really does happen in its time.

Life Hack #1

Try the One-Minute Rule. If any task can take one minute or less, then do it immediately. Making the bed, tidying your desk, washing your breakfast cup can all be done in less than a minute. If you do them instantly, then you barely notice them as a task, but leaving them can create a monumental, and quite literal pile of dishes by Friday! This theory is nothing new; the old proverb *"a stitch in time saves nine"* was first recorded in writing in 1723. Do something small now before is becomes something large and unmanageable.

Life Hack #2

What can you create in one minute or less that will last forever? How about a moment and sensation for someone else that might last a lifetime? It is so easy to do, I literally just did it, between writing Life Hacks. I messaged someone who was on my mind. *"Hi there, good morning on this fabulous Friday, I just wanted to say thanks, you're doing an amazing job and I really appreciate all you are doing."* It is really that simple, go and try it...

He has made everything beautiful in its time. He has also set eternity in the human heart; yet no one can fathom what God has done from beginning to end.

Ecclesiastes 3:11

#34

Moderation is everything

"Only actions give life strength; only moderation gives it charm."

Jean Paul (1763-1825)
German actor.

"Moderation is the silken string running through the pearl chain of all virtues."

Joseph Hall (1574-1656)
English bishop, satirist, and moralist, tending always to the middle ground in all he did.

"Everything in moderation, including moderation."

Oscar Wilde (1854-1900)
Irish poet and playwright.

Moderation is a very interesting concept, and clearly something Ewald valued enough to have even mentioned it. To be honest it's not something I've ever given much thought to, having lived and worked for most of my life at 'full throttle.' I have to say, I'm very much on the side of Oscar Wilde on this one, but let's explore how moderation can work for us and where its place fits into looking after our bodies, where there are clear benefits.

We live in a world of excess. Take a look around at the mall next time you go shopping, and if you don't notice, then the statistics speak for themselves. Here we go: *"South Africa is amongst the countries with the highest overweight and obesity rates. According to the 2016 national survey, 68% of women and 31% of men are either overweight or obese, while 13% of children under the age of 5 are overweight."* (SA Government Office of Statistics website)

In ranking for obesity South Africa rates as follows on the world list for; Woman - 25/200; Men - 131/200; and Combined - 55/200. (www.data.worldobesity.org/rankings/) Which in turn leads to increased rates of type 2 diabetes, cardiovascular diseases, hypertension, and cancer, increased risk of miscarriage, pre-eclampsia, induced labour, and women are less likely to breastfeed. Clearly, what we consume in calories for food AND drink is directly related to the obesity rates, and a lack of moderation. We are generally living a life of food AND drink excess. Why the capitalised AND? Well, guess what? - alcohol carries a high proportion of calories and where does South Africa rank on the world Health Organisation list of alcohol consumption? - 25/200. Clearly again, moderation would work here too, and save lives. In 2016, 9 760 deaths in South Africa were attributed to alcohol consumption. In 2021, 3 million people died from alcohol consumption, which is 5,3% of all deaths worldwide.

Are you consuming anything to excess? Passed the food intake test, did we? Good for you, well done! Please take out your cell phone and check the 'screen time' for yesterday and last week? Yikes! Mine even has 'Pickups', relating to the number of times I have picked-up the phone! My stats are; daily average; 111 pickups and average daily screentime 7 hours! Wow that's bad! Hope your numbers are lower? This modern-day excess is also creating issues both socially, as our children fall prey to bad influences, and physically on our bodies, as they start to show signs of "tech-neck." Poor cell phone posture of the neck always tilting downwards towards the screen causes undue pressure on the spine and many people suffer from pain there and it can result in a permanently distorted posture. What else might you be consuming to excess which might be bad for you? Only you know but check the list coming up.

Life Hack #1

What are you consuming to excess which might be considered an addiction, and not a moderate consumption. Time for a quick life-style audit. Here is a list of the world Top Ten Addictions in Modern Society. (www.caminorecovery.com/)

- Coffee (Safe Zone: <5 cups per day or 600 milligrams).
- Tobacco and Nicotine (Safe Zone: Zero intake).
- Alcohol (Safe Zone: <14 units over 7 days).
- Sex Addiction (Safe Zone: Zero for pornography).
- Illegal or prescribed drugs (Safe Zone: for illegal drugs: Zero intake).
- Gambling (Safe Zone: <failing to meet regular financial obligations).

- The Internet/Social Media (Safe Zone: You can probably use it less!).
- Video Gaming (Safe Zone: <2-3 hours per day).
- Food (Safe Zone: If you're obese and unhealthy consider reducing).
- Work (Safe Zone: Sensible "Work/Life Balance" or <8 productive hours per day).

Life Hack #2

We did the audit, which is a good first step. I think most of us over-consume on one of them somewhere, unless you're a saint. Time to make a plan to cut out or cut down - and only you can do that. Apart from the obvious addictions, in my BSR practice I see physical, mental and chemical stresses in client's bodies, from the following; *"an over-reliance on prescribed drugs"* - they tell me they don't 'feel right' about it, the internet and computer overuse leading to bad posture, teenage video gaming, again leading to bad posture, and lastly workaholism. Some folks are just addicted to work and it is literally killing them. For this life hack, you have to write your own homework question and answer it too!

Let your moderation be known unto all men. The Lord is at hand.

Philippians 4:5

#35

The body has the strictest discipline

"Pain is inevitable, suffering is optional."

Buddhist Proverb.

"The body shuts down when it has too much to bear; goes its own way quietly inside, waiting for a better time, leaving you numb and half alive."

Jeanette Winterton (1959-present)
English author.

"While burnout obviously has something to do with stress, overdoing things, not being centred, and not listening to yourself or your body, one of the deepest contributors to burnout, I believe, is the deep disappointment of not living up to your true calling, which is to help."

Jenn Bruer
American youth counsellor and a retired foster mum of 18 years on her own path to burn-out recovery.

It was Ewald's belief that, *"When the body starts disciplining you, it is the strictest discipline on earth."* The strictest of disciplines means that something inside us is pre-programmed to kick in; reactions such as a fight-or-flight, freeze, rest and digest can be triggered from a steady build-up of physical and emotional stress. Often this results in burn-out, which the World Health Organisation (WHO) classifies as *"a syndrome that stems from an occupation phenomenon."* This condition is a syndrome, not a medical diagnosis, and caused by *"chronic workplace stress that has not been successfully managed,"* according to the WHO.

As with many disciplinary processes we experience, there are stages our body goes through before really shutting down by burning out, as the strictest, and last resort. Like most of these disciplinary processes, the act of punishment occurs with the aim of improvement, recovery, and moving on, they are not punitive. It is a remedial action designed to make you better, not a punishment. The body is programmed to your benefit and always works in your favour and for your benefit, not to your detriment. Your own body, generally, cannot do you harm.

There are physical and emotional stages before burn-out and the body is given signs, which we often ignore. Listening to our body we covered in a previous wisdom (Wisdom #25). Much like disciplining anyone, the body's early warning admonishments are mild, small niggles, and aches and pains which we often ignore. We often fail to test or screen our bodies, as recommended and think it will go away. Later this discipline might escalate to major pains, severe headaches, repetitive infections, and we either tough them out or remedies fail to resolve them. Now of course, would be a good time to discover BSR, and we see many clients suffering these long-term issues in a continuous ache and pain scenario. Conversely, we see many who miss the opportunity and are in burn-out, when the journey to recovery may take rather longer. Pain is a disciplinary tool, telling us something is wrong, and a remedy at the same time signalling to the body it must act to repair us. Pain is one of the most important disciplinary tools our body has to survive. As students of Ewald's learned *"There is no healing without feeling."*

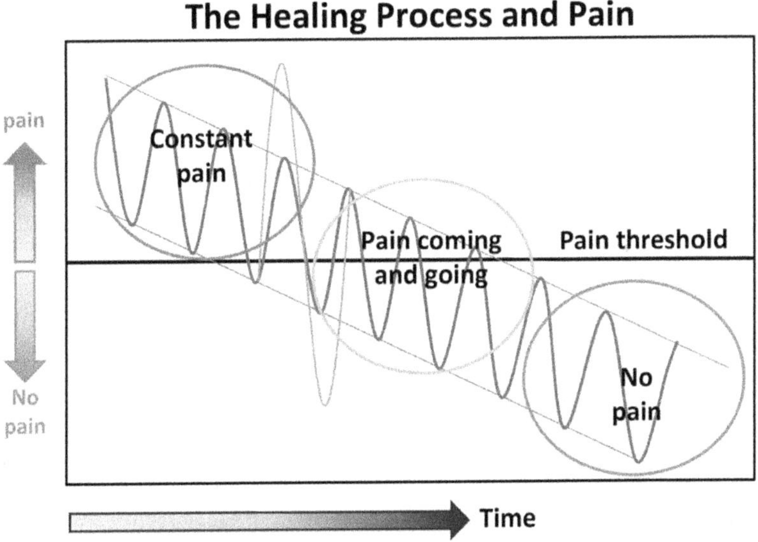

Life Hack #1

How to avoid the 'strictest of disciplines' and burn-out!

- Recognise the signs of stress.
- Set work and social boundaries.
- Have a healthy work-life balance.
- Prioritise self-care - mask-on first! (Wisdom #22)

- Exercise the body, mind, and soul.
- Take breaks regularly in all activities.
- Have support networks for both work and family groups.

(Originally from www.medicalnewstoday.com/articles/preventing-burnout)

"No, I discipline my body and make it my slave, so that after I have preached to others, I myself will not be disqualified."

1 Corinthians 9:27

#36

Resonate with yourself

"In this world, everything has a pulse or a vibration. This sound is unique to each living or non-living thing and in itself creates a music that no-one can hear. I believe that this has a very powerful resonance with, and a deep effect on, our lives."

Mike Oldfield (1953-present)
English retired musician, songwriter, and producer best known for his debut studio album Tubular Bells.

"I believe that in every person is a kind of circuit which resonates to intellectual discovery, and the idea is to make that resonance work."

Carl Sagan (1934-1996)
American astronomer, planetary scientist, and science communicator. His best-known scientific contribution is his research on the possibility of extra-terrestrial life.

What exactly is resonance? Here is a definition: *'Resonance is the occurrence of a vibrating object causing another object to vibrate at a higher amplitude. Resonance happens when the frequency of the initial object's vibration matches the resonant frequency or natural frequency of the second object.'* (www.study.com/). Every object has natural frequency at which it tends to vibrate or resonate - even inanimate solid objects such as a table and chair. More importantly, human beings also have a resonant frequency, at around 5 Hz, one Hertz being one cycle or vibration per second. However, in recent years, an indirect method has been proposed which appears to increase the resonant frequency to approximately 10 Hertz. But we wouldn't notice, would we? Also this is an average and various organs and body parts resonate at different frequencies. Such as the spinal column at 8 Hz; the brain has three resonant frequencies at 13,9, 14,2, and 14,3 Hertz; hands and arms at 20-70 Hz; and the jaw at 100-200 Hz. We are one resonating, vibrating being in a resonating world!

You can set or lower your own resonant frequency which tends to mirror your breathing rhythm. Slow breathing at a certain frequency of around 5-6 breaths per minute, steadies your resonant frequency and triggers a strong psychological heart rate response. On the inhale, the heartbeat speeds up and on the exhale it slows down, leading to a high Heart Rate Variability (HRV) and trains the Autonomic Nervous System (ANS) to be more adaptable (Max Frenzel PhD). In short, this means it helps prepare the body to cope with external or environmental stresses and threats, as well as returning the body to a resting state afterward.

The earth's resonant frequency, is around 7,83 Hertz, and it surrounds all living things on the planet. Scientific studies show that humans reach their ultimate potential for health and wellness when they resonates with this frequency. This is called the Schumann Resonance. Staying synchronised with the Earth's natural frequency can positively affect physical and mental health and daily performance and promote overall well-being. The natural resonance between humans and the earth has been severely interrupted by modern technology. Since the advent of electricity, our bodies have been increasingly bombarded with a broad spectrum of electromagnetic waves, from our electricity supply to the latest 5G cell phone technology. This interference may negatively affect the body's immune system, energy levels, and sleep quality. It could be one of the reasons why so many people often feel stressed and anxious. That said, there is currently no evidence from scientific research to suggest that low level-electromagnetic fields are harmful to human health.

All our gatherings in the BSR community begin with a 'loving thought'; for others, you might want to pray, that's OK, too. Invoking a higher power to assist can never be a bad thing, adding them into the team is a great idea! It's also perfectly acceptable, as Ewald considered, that to, *"Hold a loving thought for YOURSELF"* is also a good thing to do. Either way, the thought and moment of calmness, either in a group setting or by yourself, sets the heart to beat slower, and more coherently, especially if you add some slower and more consistent breathing.

Life Hack #1

Sleep is one of the most precious and healthy activities we do. I see an increasing number of clients struggling with good quality sleep. Sleep hygiene may be something to consider if you are struggling. One of the areas I suggest is to turn off all devices where you sleep. Better NOT to have a TV in the bedroom, but make sure its fully turned off for sleep. Likewise, and more importantly, set the cell phone on the bedside table to 'airplane' mode and the wi-fi turned off, this should minimise any potential electromagnetic interference to sleep, if it worries you.

Life Hack #2

Self-resonance is really about being true to yourself. There is a whole raft of things you can do to know and be yourself, and we covered the question *"Who are you?"* already. If you have already done that work revisit it. Knowing what makes you tick is part of achieving your own self-resonance. Now add the question *"What makes me happy?"* Doing the daily things that really please our inner selves, makes us resonant optimally. You are the only custodian of your happiness; you cannot let your happiness depend on others. Being happy also sends out the 'happiness resonance' to others too. Imagine all your happiness resonance bouncing around affecting others...

Peace I leave with you; my peace I give you. I do not give to you as the world gives. Do not let your hearts be troubled and do not be afraid.

John 14:27

#37

The heart knows

"Nature never did betray the heart that loved her."

William Wordsworth (1770-1850)
English Romantic poet who, with Samuel Taylor Coleridge, helped to launch the Romantic Age in English literature.

"The best and most beautiful things in the world cannot be seen or even touched - they must be felt with the heart."

Helen Keller (1880-1968)
American author, disability rights advocate, political activist, and lecturer.

"Your vision will become clear only when you can look into your own heart. Who looks outside, dreams; who looks inside, awakes."

Carl Jung (1875-1961)
Swiss psychiatrist, psychotherapist, psychologist, and pioneering evolutionary theorist who founded the school of analytical psychology.

At around 22 days after conception, and before the thinking brain has developed in the womb, the heart starts to beat. It continues to beat and does not stop until we die. No brain memory or activity starts off the pumping action. Even when we're adults the heart can beat on its own without signals from the brain. As long as there is enough oxygen, your heart can continue to beat even when it is separated from your body. The heart has its own electrical impulses to achieve all this. Ewald believed and said, *"The heart knows in advance what is happening."*

We have already examined the concept of the 'heart brain' and it being our emotional centre. At least metaphorically, the heart represents our emotional being. However, the heart's brain is a complex network of neurons, axons, proteins, neurotransmitters, and supporting cells similar to those in the actual brain. This complex circuitry enables it to act independently of the cranial brain; to learn, remember, and even feel and sense. The physical heart therefore, has extensive afferent connections (or nerve fibre paths) linked directly to the brain and can modulate perception and emotional experience. Our hearts really may 'know things' before the brain. There are more nerve impulses sent from the heart to the brain than vice versa. The heart is more than just a pump, as many believe.

We can actually use the power of the heart and its emotional feelings to change the world with 'happy heart-centred emotions'. Research carried out by the HeartMath® Institute, and using positive heart coherence, in groups around the world at a single moment, affected the earth's resonance at those locations. According to the Institute *"Large numbers of people creating heart-centred states of love and compassion will generate a more coherent field environment that can benefit others and help offset society's current fear and incoherence."* Love and loving feelings, from the heart (others might call that a prayer) really can make a difference, to our own environment, family and friends.

No one, however, is saying that the heart knows best. As we have considered there are three 'intelligences' at work when we react to or make decisions in our life. The heart, the brain, and the gut, and depending on your character type one may be the predominant boss of the other two. Do you run on instinct?, let the logic of situations dictate? or are you more prone to let the heart lead?, with all its emotive power and emotional weaknesses. Either way, the heart seems to be somewhat more intelligent than we usually think, and also ahead of the decision game!

Life Hack #1

Heart Lock-In® Technique is a way to activate positive heart-based emotions to reduce stress in your body.

Step 1
Focus your attention in the area of the heart, place your hand on your heart, feel your heartbeat. Imagine your breath is flowing in and out of your heart or chest area, breathing a little slower and deeper than usual.

Step 2
Activate and sustain a loving, positive feeling such as appreciation, care or compassion. You might say those words in your head *"Thank you for..."* and smile too.

Step 3
Radiate that renewing feeling to yourself and others. Radiating is

best done on the exhale when you can say in your head *"Sending you gratitude for…"*(https://www.heartmath.com/)

Above all else, guard your heart,
for everything you do flows from it.

Proverbs 4:23

#38

Honour your body

"Respect your body when it's asking for a break. Respect your mind when its seeking rest. Honour yourself when you need a moment for yourself."

Author unknown.

"Take care of your body. It's the only place you have to live."

Jim Rohn (1964-2009)
American entrepreneur, author, and motivational speaker who wrote numerous books.

"Honour your body. Keep it in good shape. It is the most important physical tool that you have. Exercise is the meditation of the body. It allows you to feel Oneness with all of Life."

Neale Donald Walsch (1943-present)
American actor, screenwriter, speaker, and author of the series Conversations with God.

The infrequently used word, 'honour' may need some revision and explaining in this case. The meaning of honour, really means *'to respect, have gratitude for or to hold something in reverence or high regard'* (Oxford Languages). In honouring your body, it is the concept of your body being a temple, a place of worship and reverence. Ever walked into a large cathedral or mosque and had that feeling of awe and greatness, especially if they are grand and ornate? I am sure you talked in a whisper and respected the guides, as they explained the building to you. There may have been certain rituals you had to do to respect the ethos of the temple, take your shoes off, remove hats or to keep heads covered etc. This is the concept we should be applying to our own bodies.

We usually consider ourselves the owners of our bodies - it is my body and my space. In reverence and gratitude, we might consider that we are only the custodians of our bodies for a brief time, and that the gift of creation and the inevitability of death belongs to the higher divine power. If we thought more like this, we might take better care of it, but generally we do not. By taking care of your own body, the correlation is that you are also honouring the divine being that created you. If you were made to a plan then we believe, it is to His likeness. The concept that He is omnipresent (everywhere at all times) means that we also contain the divine in one huge divine entity as in - our body, our group, the human race.

Strange then that we live in a world where our bodies are regularly degraded or exploited on many levels. From body shaming to human trafficking our bodies are often seen as assets to be wantonly used and exploited. Industries, cultures, and business sectors often force us to do very irreverent things to our bodies, such as; carry heavy weights, sitting for long hours at a desk, ladies wearing high heels in the sales team or to smile to customers all day long. These are not 'temple-like', honourable things to be doing with our bodies, and generally cause a discord or stress in maintaining the temple's equilibrium. All these demands I have noted from my clients, when we talk about occupational stress, and the effects on the body. Employers consider your bodies or you, as their 'greatest asset', but often refer to you impersonally as Human Capital, and certainly not as any type of temple! Here are three areas to consider for better self-worship.

Life Hack #1

If you are an office worker and spend hours at the computer, it's time to check your workspace, and the posture you adopt at your computer. There are lots of diagrams on the internet of how to set up your workstation for the best possible seating arrangement and comfort and to attain the best sitting posture. If you only have a laptop, buy a large screen and keyboard to plug in. Better still, encourage your employer to do a risk assessment for your workstation and buy a large screen for you! Laptops and their tiny screens are causing a great deal of poor posture in offices and for homeworking.

Life Hack #2

One third of your life you spend sleeping in a bed: time to check your mattress. The average spring mattress lasts for 6-10 years (15 years max.) - when was the last time you changed it? If you have a memory foam mattress it's a little better with a life span of 10-15 years. I encourage my clients to review their mattress if they have bad backs or experience poor sleeping, and to invest in a good memory-foam mattress. All part of self-care and honouring your temple.

Life Hack #3

Finally, for all the sporty, exercise types, time to look at; fit - form - and function.

Fit - Do you have properly fitting equipment, such as running shoes or had a professional bike fitting? If not, time to change the shoes or get a fitment done by a pro.

Form - The way you perform any exercise or sport must always be correct. What is your running gait like, how are you lifting weights at the gym or is your golf-swing the best it can be? Get someone professional to assist and observe and make suggestions for improvement.

Function - This comprises the frequency and intensity of your activity. Are you doing too much too often, with little rest? Review your exercise schedule and adjust to a more sensible level as required. Your body is already telling you if you're doing too much.

Don't you know that you yourselves are God's temple and that God's Spirit dwells in your midst? If anyone destroys God's temple, God will destroy that person; for God's temple is sacred, and you together are that temple.

1 Corinthians 3:16-17

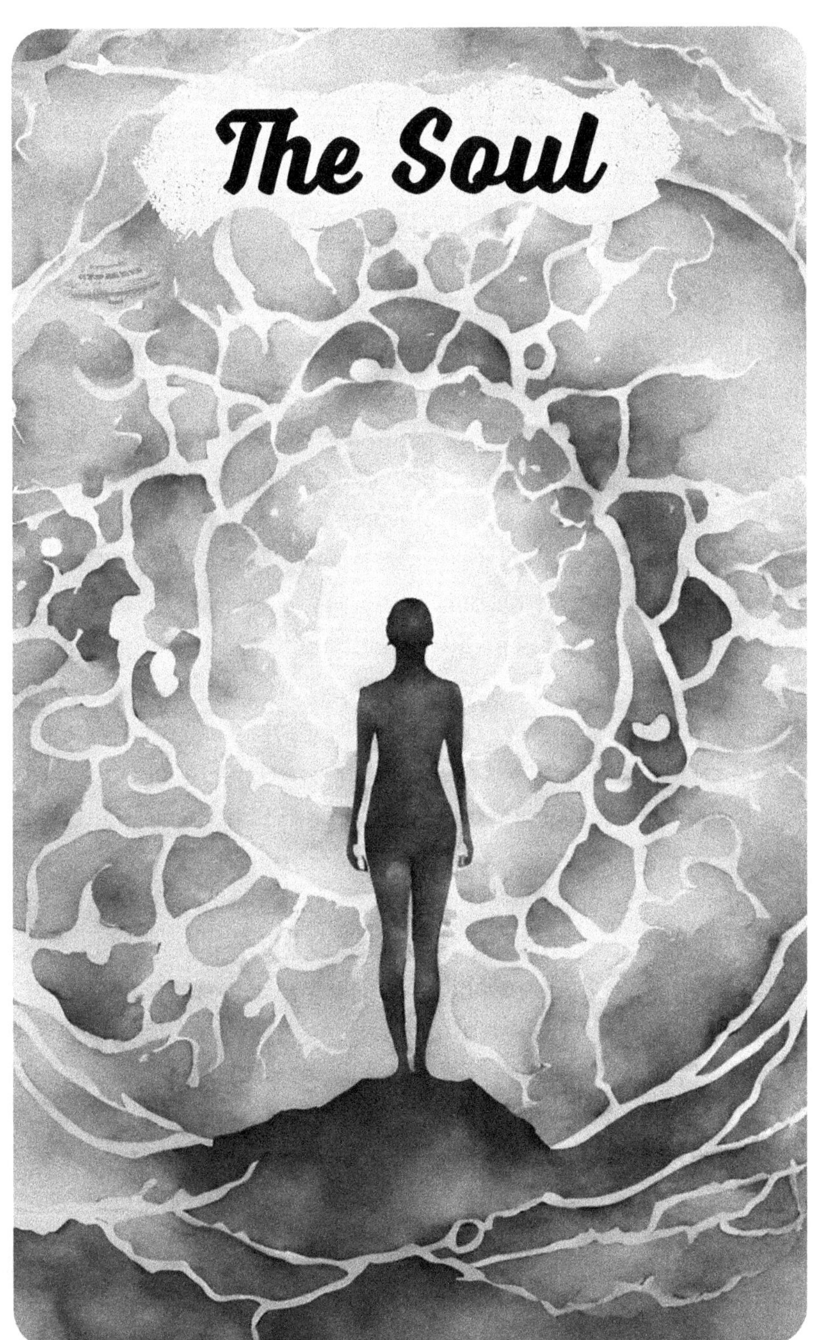
The Soul

The concept of a soul speaks of your inner-life, or life-force, in relation to your own experiences; your mind, your heart, and your imagination. It also speaks to your thoughts, desires, passions, and dreams. Not to be confused with Spirit, which talks to the higher power, the divine entity, otherwise known as God by many. This higher power is both above us and around us in the heavenly and omnipresent way, but also it is part of us, inside us. It speaks to your faith, belief, hope, love, character, and perseverance.

Ewald used to say, "*We are spiritual beings having a physical experience.*" Many people have that belief, as I do. We come from somewhere to earth for physical experiences and return to wherever we came from. The soul is that part of you that survives after death and goes someplace else. Heaven or hell, if you believe in both or maybe only one. This is, of course, not a new concept. Humankind has always had a concept of another life, a spirit world, or 'afterlife', a greater and more powerful place than the terrestrial world. Taking Ewald's quote to the next level would suggest the spirit world is the real world and the terrestrial world is the one we merely transit though for "physical experiences."

There is a soul within all of us and part of a spirit entity available to us, although not everyone chooses to tap into the latter. I understand these to be a given for every human, but you can only tap into their capability and power if you believe in them. I had a client once tell me after the first session *"This is just too light a technique for me, it's never going to work."* If you don't have belief in something then you're already starting on the back foot. As much as you meet some people who seem to be soulless, it is really in their body somewhere. It is probably hiding with their denied spirituality. I have seen many a non-believer find the need for something or someone larger and more powerful than themselves in times of crisis. When you first feel the pain of death for a loved one, a family member or military colleague, then you will really want there to be a place where they have gone. *"She's in a better place"* and *"May his soul rest in peace"*, we say are platitudes, and ones we have constructed to feel that a loved one is still there, still with us, and not quite entirely gone.

Someone still being there and around in a spirit form after death is a very common belief, and especially so in African cultures. You might call it ancestor worship, which tends to be at odds with Christian beliefs, but it is a belief in African cultures. It was never real to me until I came to Africa. Maybe you have to have an experience to become a true believer. Here's my brief experience of the afterlife if you need to know where I'm coming from?

During my redundancy phase before I became a BSR practitioner I did a semi-professional photography course. The culmination of that was a portfolio and a photo-journalism piece where I had the option to visit a sangoma in my wife's township of Daveyton, just east of Johannesburg. I jumped at the chance. The aim was to take a few images, have a reading and interview the lady sangoma. The reading of course was the most interesting part. She shook her bag of assorted bones and bits and pieces and tossed them randomly on the mat between us on the floor and proceeded to tell me my life story, in terms of health and wellness. The part which stuck a very deep chord was when she stated, *"You've been hearing noises in your house."* I had indeed heard noises. Only a few months previously, I had chased a noise all the way around my house from room to room, never finding it. *"It's your sister-in-law, she's happy you're around and back in South Africa."*

Zandile had died tragically about 4 years previously, and was very close to my wife and I. What I never told the Sangoma was that day I heard the noises; I believe I was physically touched by her too. I was sweeping the floor and felt a clear tap on my back, I thought it was my son playing and ignored it. It came again, tap, tap, and I exclaimed *"Hey Mandla!"* and spun around, expecting to find him. There was no-one. I dashed from room to room, chasing a noise, but there was no-one. No-one downstairs, my son was deeply asleep upstairs. I checked, believe you me I checked. For a time, it freaked me out until someone I'd never met before told me who it was, by looking at a mess of bones and stuff on the floor. I've had a few similar experiences.

How to explain the soul and the spirit is never easy, but for me it's real. From my experiences, it's very real and I am sure that those who don't believe in it can find a logical way to rationalise it away. I am fine with that, so long as my belief and my experiences are also respected. In the final section of the book, you will have to 'come as you are' in your belief of soul and spirit and 'take what you need and disregard the rest.' There will never be an aim to convert or convince, just for me to highlight the final few of Ewald's wisdoms I placed in soul domain.

#39

Develop a sense of joy

"He who laughs most, learns best."

John Cleese (1939-present)
English actor, comedian, screenwriter, producer, and presenter.

"If you carry joy in your heart, you can heal any moment."

Carlos Santana (1947-present)
American guitarist, best known as a founding member of the rock band Santana.

"A thing of beauty is a joy forever: its loveliness increases; it will never pass into nothingness."

John Keats (1795-1821)
English poet of the second generation of Romantic poets. His poems had been in publication for less than four years when he died of tuberculosis at the age of 25.

Joy is fun, and it's the second tenet in my own list of life purposes after trusting in God. Having joy and fun in your life, brings with it a unique feeling, an inner peace and contentment. This is the best way I find to describe it. In general, I've had an exciting and joyful life so far, not that there were no hard times, or things I regret. There certainly are a few regrets, but you cannot let these change you or bring you down. They really do have to become water under the bridge, so long as you learned a lesson or two along the way. No-one is responsible for your joy and happiness but you, and own it you must.

While happiness can come from the mind and doing things that make you feel happy, joy, for me, is really a soul activity. The former comes and goes as we do things and meet people in our daily lives, that makes us happy over a period of time, whereas joy is an inner soulful feeling. Joy always happens in the moment, spontaneously, when we do something joyful, such as a walk in the sun, listen to a memorable song, pet a puppy or eat a favourite food. It is actually much easier to find joy in our lives and trigger it, than it is to find longer term happiness. Research has found that these moments of joy often have a 'halo effect', where their impact reaches far beyond the moment of joy itself. In many ways, those little moments of joy add up to more than the sum of their parts. Over time, their cumulative effects may lead to greater through life happiness. Soulful joy also feeds the mind and the body too. (www.aestheticsofjoy.com/).

Joy, unsurprisingly, is also good for our health. Studies have shown that there are positive links between the feelings of joy and physical wellbeing. Joyful people have been shown to have lower cortisol, inflammation, and blood pressure, with some researchers believing that these effects may help reduce the risk of cardiovascular disease, and even help us live longer. Experiencing genuine joyful emotions is also contagious, it encourages joy in others, and guess what?, it is attractive to others too. In studies, people rate smiling faces of average attractiveness as more appealing than non-smiling faces of above-average looks. But take care, a fake smile isn't going to work! Joy brings on what is known as a Duchenne smile, discovered by French anatomist Duchenne de Boulogne in 1862, it is an involuntary one, that involves the orbicularis oculi muscles - the ones around the eyes. Yes we really do smile with our eyes, so best not to Botox out those joyful 'laughter lines!' as they radiate our joy to others.

As Ewald used to say "*Joy is oneness.*" And it is contagious, and spreads like a ripple on a pond.

Life Hack #1

What do you love the most that gives you that daily fix of joy? For me it's the combination of a sundowner while I cook dinner and listening to my favourite music. The ultimate 'me time' with some creativity of the recipe (or not!) and of course a giving element for those who need to be fed. For you, it might be reading, gardening, exercise or just listening to music.

Life Hack #2

Find joy in your daily life and in the mundane. Everyone in my house has headphones on, and while it's difficult to hold a conversation at times, cleaning the house or washing the dishes becomes that much more joyful with music. Likewise, turning something into a game can be fun. Clients lying face down on my BSR bed use a tissue for hygiene purposes. When they get up, I scrunch it into a ball and throw it into the waste-paper basket - basketball style. When I'm feeling lucky, I throw it over my shoulder. I even keep the score, and once got a *"Good shot!"* remark from one client.

A joyful heart is good medicine,
but a crushed spirit dries up the bones.

Proverbs 17:22

#40

Your beliefs determine your reality

"Fake it until you make it."

Simon & Garfunkel Lyric to "Fakin' it" (1967)
Also a mantra while perfecting the BSR technique at our Academy!

"I have learned that as long as I hold fast to my beliefs and values - and follow my own moral compass - then the only expectations I need to live up to are my own."

Michelle Obama (1964-present)
American attorney and author who served as the first lady of the United States.

"I feel like that's my foundation and my roots, what I believe in - no matter where life takes me, I'll always be the same guy and same person at heart."

Morgan Wallen (1993-present)
American country pop singer who competed in the sixth season of The Voice.

Let's start with the elephant in the room 'Faking it till we make it' doesn't sound too genuine does it? Otherwise known as *"acting as if you already have it - in an act to get yourself to the point of believing"*. As Rhona Byrne, suggests in *The Secret, "Start make-believing. Be like a child, and make-believe. Act as if you have it already. As you make-believe, you will begin to believe you have received."* In my early writing career (I'm even faking it now calling it a career!), I called myself an author, even before my first printed book was launched. I had a dream, I knew I was going to do it, so I pre-empted the publication somewhat. I created reality out of a belief. Once you make it - no need to fake it of course! Self-belief is crucial in achieving dreams, and they originate from the soul.

A belief is something you hold to be true, and our 'belief system' starts to acquire information from the moment we are born. Shaped and codified by our upbringing, both nurture and nature play a role in how we see the world and most importantly how the world sees us. They might also be called norms and values, and form the set of rules that guide us in achieving what we want to, and is covered in another wisdom. What we believe in, is rooted in our past, and in our early developmental years.

The most important connection however, in terms of belief, and the one that is most fundamental, is that to our spiritual belief system. That is if you have one, some don't and some choose not to believe in anything at all. However, practising a belief system may offer benefits such as a sense of comfort, a purpose in life, and a connection to others. This can be especially beneficial during challenging times. Also, beliefs can affect the healing process and improve quality of life, the power of prayer and a divine entity can be a tremendous asset to us. If you practise a belief, and your commitment grows, it may also turn into a set of values you use in every-day life. Belief systems can be a great motivation and provide a framework for life and growth, but often it literally does take a leap of faith. While it's good to have a questioning mind in a belief system, not everything can be explained at all times.

Life Hack #1

Clarity helps in aligning your belief system with your aspirations. Reflect on your existing beliefs. Be specific and write down your goals, spiritual or otherwise. Identify any limiting beliefs that may hinder your progress. Specific spiritual journaling can be a helpful tool for this reflection. Replace any of the limiting beliefs you might have with positive affirmations, which can alter your refreshed reality.

Life Hack #2

Commit to continual spiritual growth. In a hectic world our belief system can be the one that suffers first, either when we're too busy or not in need of support quite so much. Consider reading faith books more, attending more (events or courses) or seek some sort of spiritual mentor.

Do not let your hearts be troubled.
You believe in God; believe also in me.

John 14:1

#41

No self-judgement

"If you are your authentic self. There is no competition."

Lotte Mooij (Not Known)
Dutch BSR Practitioner, Class of 2015 and classmate of the author.

"Self-judgment. It's like this little voice inside our head that critiques every action, decision or thought we have. But here's the thing: this constant judgment of ourselves creates our own suffering. It's an unhappiness of our own making."

Chase Jarvis (1971-present)
American photographer, director, artist, and entrepreneur, who was CEO of CreativeLive, an on-line education platform.

"Your best changes from moment to moment, sick or well, tired or rested. Remember that you are an imperfect human being. There is no value to judging yourself."

Don Miguel Ruiz (1952-present)
Mexican author of Toltec and neo-shamanistic texts.

A good section to reiterate the quote from Don Ruiz, *"Remember that you are an imperfect human being."* Actually much of our strength, beauty, and power resides in that part we might not see as perfect. If we were made to a divine plan and likeness, you might imagine we would have been made perfect? Well take a look at any new-born baby and you're going to say, *"Awwww, he/she's perfect."* I am sure you have all done that at some time. So how do we end up so judgemental of ourselves as we progress in life? I have to tell you there is a saviour point coming. At a certain age you really do give up self-judgement; it either takes too much energy, or really you just do not care anymore of what others think. Quite a cool place to be I have to tell you!

As we have read, we're all highly individual human beings, yet 99,9% the same genetically, born pretty perfect, and now in later life well, let's say... way from perfect? Perhaps there is a better way? Instead of judging and comparing ourselves to define our current state. Clearly, some of our foibles and imperfections can be attractive to an extent, maybe even quirky - and hopefully not downright annoying! We are on a journey, developing and learning along the way, guided by our soul, influenced by spirit and belief. Sometimes in our personality and character will change, and some not. The other way to perceive this is, instead of judging ourselves, might be to just live an authentic life being true to yourself.

It is hard to imagine my good friend and classmate on the BSR Course, in 2015, would scrawl in my notebook - *"If you are your authentic self. There is no competition"*, and it be original. I love the quote, very Oscar Wilde, and I was sure attributable to someone else? Not so, all the internet references are to dates later than 2015! So, Lotte prescribes an authentic life which is judgement free, as there really is no competition. In this way, we are made perfect and there is also no comparison to who we really are. But how do we become our "authentic selves"? This means always being true and real to yourself, in that you have to live your purpose in life, honour your values and commit to your belief system. Just be you, it really is good enough.

Life Hack #1

Ban the word 'should', its loaded, negative, and a judgemental word. *"I should have gone to college"*; rather *"Going to college at that time wasn't right for me"* or *"I should be more outgoing"*; rather *"I'm much better one-on-one and really thrive in those situations."* No more 'should' - next time stop and find the positive and stop judging others or yourself. Or better still, stop the guilt-trip of self-judgement and create an opportunity... *"I could be more outgoing?"* Now it's a question with potential for something new...

Life Hack #2

Authenticity takes practice - which means it takes patience, time, and dedication to doing it. One way you can build your 'muscle of authenticity' is to take small, daily actions that align with your values. Try these in all you do:

- Be true to your word.
- Don't take anything personally.
- Have boundaries and learn to say no (nicely).
- Always do your best.

For we must all appear before the judgment seat of Christ, so that each one may receive what is due for what he has done in the body, whether good or evil.

2 Corinthian 5:10

#42

You receive what you give

"The law of attraction, states that good thinking attracts good results. Whatever you focus on, be it positive or negative, you will attract into your life."

From *The Secret*.
Rhonda Byrne (1951-present)
Australian television writer and producer.

"Whatever the mind can conceive it can achieve."

William Clement Stone (1902-2002)
American businessman, philanthropist, and self-help book author.

"What you radiate outward in your thoughts, feelings, mental pictures and words, you attract into your life."

Catherine Ponder (1927-present)
American minister and founder of Unity Church Worldwide and author of several New Thought books focused on the theme of prosperity.

If you can imagine your body as a transmitter, both in the soulful and mindful domain then quite definitely the Law of Attraction applies, (as purported in the bestseller *The Secret*) - like attracts like, in this case. If you're positive then positive things generally happen, if you're negative then you're going to attract negative things. The other two Laws are; nature hates a vacuum; and the present is always perfect, are also amazing propositions.

Whatever you're putting out there is being reflected and maybe even magnified by the environment you're in, right back to you. But these are not scientific laws like the Law of Gravity. They are belief, soul-based laws. As Henry Ford (1863-1947) said *"Whether you think you can, or you think you can't - you're right."* I am not sure why anyone would want to put out negativity, other than the media, but a lot of people seem to. I've seen too many people when faced with new ideas, choices or opportunities to give charitably say "What if it doesn't..." The negative nay-sayers will always be there, to which I usually respond back "What if it does...?"

The second law also applies in this instance. This is a science-based law: *"The second Law of Attraction is based on the laws of thermodynamics in that it is impossible to create a completely empty space because atoms are always bouncing around and immediately try to fill an empty space."* (www.lifecoach.com/) Creating or giving space to a situation, allows that space to be filled by something else in return. Sometimes you have to take a risk, fire that key person in the company without having a replacement, or resign from a voluntary post and not find a replacement. Nature and the organisations concerned will always fill the space. It is the same in all the spaces in our life; take a look at your workspace, diary, kitchen cupboards, wardrobe and sock drawer. Clear them out and see what happens. The same might also be true of some emotions we are investing in, it's usually in too many areas, perhaps it's time for an emotional audit and clear out here too?

Life Hack #1

Create space, and clean your clutter out! Start with the physical space that is causing you or your family the most amount of grief. For me that would be the garage. I inherited a 'Keep it just in case' post-World War Two mentality from my Granddad and his shed, it was packed with everything - just in case. Well, #MeToo! Here I'm always fighting the law of 'If you throw it away you'll need it now Law.' But fight it you have to, don't keep your school books from 20 years ago, you really don't need them.

Life Hack #2

Lazy hack this one, you could find new areas to donate your time, talent and treasures into preferably, but this works equally as well. Try to give more of whatever you're currently giving. Turn the dial up on your giving and see what happens, usually giving more will return more several fold.

Do not be deceived, God is not mocked; for whatever a man sows, that he will also reap. For he who sows to his flesh will of the flesh reap corruption, but he who sows to the Spirit will of the Spirit reap everlasting life.

Galatians 6: 7-8

#43

Pay attention to your dreams

"Don't let your dreams be dreams."

Jack Johnson (1975-present)
American singer-songwriter and environmental activist.

"Dreams come a size too big so that we can grow into them."

Josie Bissett (1970-present)
American television actress.

"The biggest adventure you can take is to live the life of your dreams."

Oprah Winfrey (1954-present)
American talk show host, television producer, actress, author, and media proprietor.

I love this definition by John C Maxwell *"A dream is an inspiring picture of the future that energises your mind, will, and emotions, empowering you to do everything you can to achieve it."* It started me on my own dream journey to be a published author. Maxwell's book *Put Your Dream to the Test*, became my sole (and soulful) guide to achieving my dream, which worked to the extent, I am now living my dream to the fullest, at least for this phase of my life. Next step is to revisit the book I once used for the next BIG DREAM! In a life without limits, why just have one? Time for the next one.

By their nature, dreams are BIG and aspirational, when Martin Luther King Jr. proclaimed in his 1963 speech *"I have a dream."* His dream, as he proclaimed it would, went down in history and he proclaimed it to the whole world. So, pay attention to your dreams, they are soul felt, they usually come from deep within, and are part of your entire being. Often they sit there, untended and unloved, until one day opportunity knocks. My first dream was to work for myself. When I left the military I thought of being a self-employed consultant, the idea of controlling my own work schedule really appealed to me after a life of organisation and discipline. Then it was just too BIG and too scary, it was only when I was retrenched 8 years later, that it was finally realised. I didn't work for two years which led to me needing BSR, and that opportunistic question *"Why don't you become a practitioner?"* BIG dream and opportunity perfectly matched at just the right time! The second dream was met in a similar way, as the 10 years' worth of research filed away on my computer, came together with two and a half months of nothing to do during the COVID-19 lockdown. BIG dream again met opportunity, but this time needed an enormous amount of work to realise the dream. I had huge obstacles to overcome, but most of them only lay in my own mind, with my own fear.

Fear, is the demon 'dream-slayer' or as we say in BSR the 'kabouter'. He (sorry ladies these little guys only seem to come in the male form) and are tiny naughty, gnome-like beings in red pointy hats, who usually create havoc by 'nay-saying'. Physically, they are usually Dutch carnival characters, and metaphorically reside in all of us as self-doubt and fear. He'll probably start to nag you with - *"That dream's way too BIG for you!"* and it only get worse after that, by the end of a 'kabouter session', you won't have the skillset, time, effort, energy or money to get even half way to your dream. For me, he is my 'To Do List' guy who helps me plan what barriers I need to overcome to achieve my dream. The BIGGEST of his doubts gets the most attention, and then the next, and the next, and so on until he's run out of his naughty kabouter thoughts. First part done, plan made, and self-doubt eliminated.

Life Hack #1

Step 1; in making this dream become real, is to give it life. Write it down. My dream is to ....
.... {fill in the blanks}
If you don't do that then you end up with a 'Bucket List' - but that's only a list of experiences and achievements you most likely won't ever achieve. It's OK to have one of those too, like a reserve mini-dream list. Top of mine is to visit Cuba. There, I've told you, and now someone will ask me, *"Simon when are you visiting Cuba?"* I think it's good to get your dreams out there. The 'to share or not to share question?' is always a kabouter doubt which sneaks in, and based on insecurity. I say, give it life and proclaim it, a bit like Dr Martin Luther King Jr! All you have to do is share your dream with someone, maybe even create a Dream Team to support you, to

make your dreams come true.

Life Hack #2

Step 2; start to visualise it. Each day, and I mean each and every day, add some small detail, allow the mental picture of your dream to grow. Dreams need to take on a form. In this step, start to research and collect detail. Find someone, or a group of people, who have already achieved your dream. Start to follow them on social media, join mail lists, buy books, read and learn how your dream works. Your dream is BIG, or at least it should be, but someone, somewhere has most likely achieved your dream for themselves already. It's OK to have a support team, now is a good time to create that Dream Team.

Life Hack #3

Step 3; Do something towards achieving your dream! You should have a 'kabouter list' by now that you've already turned into some list or plan and files with some research material. Now is the time to take action and eat that BIG DREAM elephant in the room, one small task or action at a time. Every day do something positive towards achieving your next dream. Now it's time to go back to my next BIG DREAM File, and dust it off...

"We both had dreams," they answered, "but there is no one to interpret them." Then Joseph said to them, "Do not interpretations belong to God? Tell me your dreams."

Genesis 40:8

#44

Intention needs to be pure

"We either live with intention or exist by default."

Kristen Armstrong (1973-present)
American cyclist and 3-times Olympic gold medallist.

"When your intentions are pure you don't lose anyone. People lose you."

Anon.

"Intention is one of the most powerful forces there is. What you mean when you do a thing will always determine the outcome. The law creates the World."

Brenna Yovanoff (1979-present)
American young-adult author.

Intention is best seen as an aim or a plan, but might also be described as a purpose or desire. You might choose a visionary whole-life intention by which you live your life or perhaps, as I did, choose a short set of life of intentions by which you guide your daily life. It is really up to you - but having intention in a singular moment provides clarity and focus, and things you do stand a better chance of success. But one intention at a time please! Be present in your moment of intent, no multi-tasking of intentions is allowed! In a life where we try to use our cell phones, hold a conversation and, in South Africa - drive a car too! Clearly nothing can be done to its most productive level!

The 'purity' clause, Ewald added, requires a singular clarity for sure, but also one with no caveats or expectations. In gold terms your intention needs to be 24 karat, the purest form of gold in its refined state. Intention is much like a prayer, given to the higher power with no caveats. If your intention is phrased as *"If I - will you?"* it probably won't work, as it is conditional. Pure intention works, but maybe not always to your expected time frame. Good things really do come to those who wait, and patience is the fuel that feeds great intention. The alternative of course, as Kristen Armstrong says, "...is life by default" and in her world the clarity and purity of intention is to do only one thing - bring home the proverbial 24-karat gold medal.

Life Hack #1

Think of each momentary intention throughout the day as a gold medal. If you focus on this with singular pure intention - see how many medals you can win at the end of the day!

Life Hack #2

Advanced intention! Try that thing you've always wanted to do but been too scared to do. With singularity of thought, a deep breath, and some modest bravery, you might just bake that souffle, ask that person out on a date or get that new job... The world is waiting for your next, new, scary intention!

Finally, brothers and sisters, whatever is true, whatever is noble, whatever is right, whatever is pure, whatever is lovely, whatever is admirable, if anything is excellent or praiseworthy, think about such things.

Philippians 4:8

#45

Your beliefs limit your achievements

"The human body has limitations. The human spirit is boundless."

Dean Karnazes (1962-present)
American ultra-marathon runner and author of Ultramarathon Man: Confessions of an All-Night Runner.

"I'm not interested in your limiting beliefs; I'm interested in what makes you limitless."

Brendon Burchard (1977-present)
American author, high-performance coach, and motivational speaker.

"Do the uncomfortable. Become comfortable with these acts. Prove to yourself that your limiting beliefs die a quick death if you will simply do what you feel uncomfortable doing."

Darren Rowse – aka ProBlogger (1972-present)
Australian blogger, speaker, consultant, and founder of several blogs and blog networks.

Our early belief system is created from our roots and our parents, and forms our early norms and values. These are defined as *"Values are important beliefs or ideals of a person in a community, serving as a motivation for action. Norms are action-guiding rules. The difference is a value is general, referring to an overall ideal, whereas a norm is concrete, specifying certain things that have to be done (or omitted)."* (www. embassy.science/).

Cultural norms come in four types and are usually passed down to people from their families, friends, and acquaintances in their social circle, from birth, but can also be learned throughout life. They are summarised as follows:

4 Types of Cultural Norms	Difference Between Types
Laws	Right versus Illegal
Folkways	Right versus Rude
Mores	Right versus Wrong
Taboos	Right versus Forbidden

Of course, the definition of "Right", though considered absolute is open to debate, as your 'rude' might not be my 'rude', and your 'wrong' might be my 'right'. It is not worth challenging the legal norms, but of course for every charge and court appearance there is a counsel for the defence to prove innocence...

In my own case, I always believed I could write a book, I had one in me since secondary school, and my two brilliant English teachers inspired me to love the written word. Then I became a miliary engineer and when I came to write my first book 50 years later, no publisher would touch it - *"It will never sell, it's too niche"* they told me. Well someone else's *"never"*, should never be a limit to you, it should always be overcome by your own belief to achieve your dream. Currently, I am writing books, 4, and 5!

Life Hack #1

Who was the last person to say, *"never"* to you? Or did your inner doubter, the kabouter, say to you *"You'll never do that?"* The word never is a real belief limitation. Write down your 'nevers', then underneath, draw two columns, and start the list; 'I will never...' in the left column; and 'How can I?' in the right column, and change that 'never' into an "I can do this"... As Nelson Mandela (1918-2013) is reputed to have said, *"It always seems impossible until it's done."*

Life Hack #2

Create a totally new belief about yourself and what you can do, something to improve the quality of your life. Remember, it's never too late to start. The new belief might start with *"I think I might be able to.."* now change it into *"I can..."* Say it out loud. It might be something new socially, removing a fear or excuse, you might have inherited a belief system you want to change, or change some societal norm imposed on you.

I can do all things through Him who strengthens me.

Philippians 4:13

#46

Never lose sight of the bigger picture

"Your vision will become clear only when you can look into your own heart. Who looks outside, dreams; who looks inside, awakes."

Carl Jung (1875-1961)
Swiss psychiatrist, psychotherapist, and psychologist.

"The challenge is not to be perfect - it is to be whole."

Jane Fonda (1937-present)
American actress and activist. Recognised as a film icon, her work spans several genres, and over six decades of film and television.

"Big picture thinkers broaden their outlook by striving to learn from every experience. They don't rest on their successes, they learn from them."

John C Maxwell (1947-present)
American author, speaker, and pastor who has written many books, primarily focusing on leadership.

We see the world through our eyes and mind, and if we treat ourselves like a camera, we can either zoom in to the detail or zoom out to the wider, more general and larger perspective. The widest of our views is considered to be our worldview, defined as: *"A collection of attitudes, values, stories and expectations about the world around us, which inform our every thought and action. Worldview is expressed in ethics, religion, philosophy, scientific beliefs and so on."*(Sire, 2004).

In essence, it is the lens through which you view both the micro (smaller part) and the macro (big picture or whole system view). The two extremes of accepted worldview are the mechanistic and the holistic. In the mechanistic view, small parts are considered piece-meal, in a disconnected or dissociated way. It is the realm of the specialist, their niche and generally their sole expertise. In medicine the oncologist, the neuro-surgeon and dermatologist reside in this space. The holistic view is one of large systems and interconnectedness, nothing is broken down to smaller elements. At its extreme, it is a systems-of-systems philosophy linking the human body to the whole universe. On earth it is the realm of the 'Butterfly Effect.' A theory offered by mathematician and meteorologist Edward Lorenz, in which he noted that the butterfly effect is derived from the example of the details of a tornado (at the exact time of formation, and the exact path taken) being influenced by minor perturbations such as a distant butterfly flapping its wings several weeks earlier. The concept is now often used outside of weather science, and can be applied in any area, where small events might cause bigger events to occur.

Ewald used to say, *"No matter how high you go and look down, there is always a bigger picture."* Meaning that there is always room for one more step back in viewing or looking or considering another viewpoint. The secret in any situation is knowing when enough 'bigger picture thinking' is really enough? Rick Tamlyn's book *Play Your Bigger Game,* has a great many tools for helping you gain this way of thinking, which many will find difficult to grasp and often down-right annoying. Let's look at two in the following Life Hacks.

Life Hack #1

Get out of your comfort zone. Staying in one place won't ever allow you to gain bigger-picture views, you need to keep moving and changing. If you're not, then your lens is stuck. Also try something new, with things that change your view of life, keep doing it until you get the T-shirt, which says, *"Been there - done that!"* Then start all over again.

Life Hack #2

Stop trying to be perfect. Wow for a Virgo zodiac sign, that is a difficult one to write, we like neat and tidy and everything in its place, all the time. Most detail-orientated people will struggle on this one, but the continual striving for perfection will hold you back from seeing the bigger picture, learn to let go of looking for the perfect plan or solution. Often the 80% fit in life will do, then move on. The 20% that you perceive as imperfect or missing, while searching for perfection, others won't even notice. Jane Fonda really was right - *"The challenge is not to be perfect - it is to be whole."*

The grass withers, the flower fades,
but the word of our God will stand forever.

Isaiah 40:8

#47

Healing comes from above-down, and inside-out

"Healing is a daily event. You can't 'go somewhere' to be healed; you must go inward to be healed. This means a daily commitment to doing the work."

Dr Nicole LePera (Not Known)
Aka the Holistic Psychologist with over 2 million Instagram followers.

"The way to control your life is to control your choice of words and thoughts. No-one thinks in your mind but you."

Louise L Hay (1926-2017)
American author of Heal Your Body: The Mental Causes for Physical Illness and the Metaphysical Way to Overcome Them.

"Nothing can cure the soul but the senses, just as nothing can cure the senses but the soul."

Oscar Wilde (1854-1900)
Irish poet and playwright

Ewald thought that *"The body's self-healing capability was God's gift to us."* After all, the joining of one egg and one sperm has all the genetic code to create one human being. Sometimes, it even divides to create multiple births! In the DNA there is all the information needed to create life and to sustain it through its self-healing capability. It is a complex bio-mechanical system that self-adjusts, and self-manages to keep us going and heal ourselves for the majority of instances. In addition, we all have the ability to believe in a higher entity to look over us and to give us guidance on our healing journey, but not all choose to accept it into their lives. I tell many of my religious clients to go away and pray about getting well. Why wouldn't you want to tap into this on your healing journey, in whatever faith you chose? This is the 'above-down' reference in Ewald's wisdom.

Belief in the higher power can also be belief in the healing modality and treatments you undertake while healing. This belief is really a positive energy, we can convert it into positive thoughts as well, through directed mediation. The heart-resonance hacks you have done already would be an example of turning the belief into heart-felt energy and directing those feelings as nerve signals back to the brain. The flow of soulful energy in this case is very much 'inside-out.' The energy might also flow out of us into the world around us. This is part of a 'vitalistic energy', or life-energy flow that goes beyond the explicable laws of physics and chemistry. Other doctrines call this Prana (Sanskrit), Life-Force Energy, Qi (Eastern) and Chi (Eastern), and are all ancient terms for the same thing. They may be referring to our soul, that part we are pretty sure exists after life has passed.

If referred to in these terms, healing is not an event we do only when we're sick, but is a daily part of sustaining life and lifestyle. Although we should not reject our trust and belief in western traditional medicine, there is so much more we ourselves can be doing on our own healing journeys. As William Shakespeare said, *"It is not in the stars to hold our destiny but in ourselves."* It also fits very well to Ewald's thoughts on healing and his teaching of the BSR principles to his students, that *"No person has ever healed another"* he used to say. As practitioners we have learnt to be part of our client's healing journey, but not as healers or the source of their healing. No, that is contained in the above-down and inside-out wisdom Ewald talks about.

Life Hack #1

Many of my clients suffer from past trauma in their lives. It is not always beneficial to revisit traumas and talk through it repeatedly as sometimes this only adds to it, re-opening old wounds. The healing from this healing hack, is to realise how we want to live, post trauma, and how we want to feel and then look at how our thoughts, beliefs, and behaviours are keeping us from living this life. I often encourage them to work with other professionals on their emotional healing journey whilst I focus on their physical one. (https://connectedtoself.com/healing-hack/)

Life Hack #2

Many of the hacks we've already covered can help you in this more soulful consideration of self-healing. So, try meditation focused on drawing down healing energy from above and allowing it to flow inside you. Maybe journal your thoughts after that and see what thoughts and actions you can take into your day to affect your healing journey. Only you will really know what you need to do.

And he said to them, "Doubtless you will quote to me this proverb, 'Physician, heal yourself.' What we have heard you did at Capernaum, do here in your hometown as well."

Luke 4:23

#48

Earn the right to tap into higher frequencies

"A real friend is one who walks in when the rest of the world walks out."

Walter Winchell (1897-1972)
American newspaper gossip columnist and radio news commentator.

"In the sweetness of friendship let there be laughter, and sharing of pleasures. For in the dew of little things the heart finds its morning and is refreshed."

Khalil Gibran (1883-1931)
Lebanese-American writer, poet, and visual artist; he was also considered a philosopher, although he himself rejected the title.

"Every friendship with God and every love between Him and a soul is the only one of its kind."

Janet Erskine Stuart (1857-1914)
English religious sister in the Roman Catholic Church who founded a number of schools.

If you believe 'higher frequencies' means that to be from the higher power, which is really a euphemism for God, then to earn that right, all you have to do is believe. Pure and simple. Ewald did believe in a God, and in divine love from above, so the right is earned by faith and belief, whatever that means for you. In earning it, you would normally have to by definition, 'receive something different by doing something or working for it.' So you earn the right through belief, trust, and communicating. Generally, in a faith-based system, 'tapping in' means some sort of communication, usually in the form of prayer or meditation. In many ways, friendship and love from God as the ultimate friend and Father, do not have to be truly earned; they are given freely and unconditionally. That higher power is always there, all you have to do is open your heart and communicate with it.

Many however, don't believe in a God at all and consider that our 'higher power' is really a higher, more spiritual part of our own human consciousness. Consciousness theories prior to the 1990s were more philosophical in nature, whereas today the studies in this field are more scientific. Although as humans, and considering our own consciousness, the domain is still largely considered subjective and impossible to study empirically. In addition, the topic has also been hijacked by mystical practitioners and has taken criticism for being too 'off-the-wall', by many in the field of human sciences.

Ewald however, was knowledgeable of work carried out by the Bob Monroe Institute, which is known to be a leading centre for the study of human consciousness. It takes a non-dogmatic experiential approach which students use to pursue their own personal exploration of human consciousness. They use sound waves to stimulate the brain during meditation, which is part of stimulating Out-of-Body Experiences (OBE) as higher human consciousness. The Institute publishes scientific papers and such topics as altered states of consciousness, and in 1994 the United States Army sent a number of students on its Gateway Programme, maybe there is some way to take your soulful consciousness, on an OBE, and journey to places in another dimension.

Life Hack #1

Some generic meditation in a quiet place each day on your own, most likely isn't going to get you to a higher level of consciousness or in a frame for deep prayer within your belief system. It is probably best to try a guided meditation program such as that by Dr Joe Dispenza (https://drjoedispenza.com/).

Fear you not; for I am with you: be not dismayed; for I am your God: I will strengthen you; yes, I will help you; yes, I will uphold you with the right hand of my righteousness.

Isaiah 41:10

#49

Stand in your own power

"If we all did the things we are capable of doing, we would literally astound ourselves."

Thomas Edison (1847-1931)
American Inventor and Businessman.

"Everything you could possibly ever want, have, or need is right here inside of you."

Kristin McGee (1973-present)
Fitness Coach.

Gold! - always believe in your soul
You've got the power to know
You're indestructible
Always believing - you are gold!

Lyrics to Gold by Spandau Ballet (1983)

The 'POWER Potential' is a capacity to take action, and to stand in it, is to take action to do it or declare it. With it comes an acceptance that who you are or what your organisation stands for, is already good enough, no validation required. Although some is always nice to have. Notice too, no-one is saying *"Sit quietly in a corner in your own power"*, it's standing, and standing tall too. You cannot be a 'shrinking violet' on this one. But power comes in many forms, no-one says you have to be Mohammed Ali. Some of the most powerful people I have ever met have been the quietest and most modest. Thinking about my list right now, very many that spring immediately to mind are women, with my own Mother right at the top of my list. I'm guessing many of you might do the same.

Power in this context has nothing at all to do with strength at all, but everything to do with "brand you", and being authentic. What do you want people to see in you? What values do you have that you want to transmit to the world? This must become your power dynamic, each and every day. You cannot be authentic during the week and take the weekend off to be someone else. Standing in your own power, is a true lifestyle activity. I think we have already accepted on our journey that you are 'The Perfect You' with no competition, and that we must accept our imperfections as part of that. Being authentic doesn't mean being infallible, in fact making mistakes and learning from them is very much part of adding to our power by learning along the way.

Ewald said *"We all have this capacity to allow more of the potential within each of us to express itself"* (Meggersee, 2007). The standing part is really the expression of the power capacity that Ewald talks about in this quote. If you want to express wisdom then you have to be wise; or if you want to have integrity then you have to show it, and so on with every quality that is YOUR POWER.

- Not mine or anyone else's, your power profile is unique to you.

Life Hack #1

Consider yourself gifted in terms of Time - One hour; Talent - One Skill; and Treasure - the worth of one large Latté coffee! (Remember its $5.46 or R100) And consider how you might give all of them away once a month to someone who is in need. It is often the act of releasing your inner power in the service of others, that allows you to better appreciate your own strength, and over time makes you stronger.

Life Hack #2

Speak your mind. Our words and intentions can be very powerful, but often we hide them for fearful reasons. There will be someone in your life who needs your honest, powerful, kind, and honest words, speaking your truth to others, is part of your authentic you 'superpower'. Often speaking the words, *"I love you, I need you, I appreciate all you do"*, are enough, because you already are enough, and somebody may need to hear and feel that too. Likewise, and if needed, *"I don't like that or its not acceptable"*, are equally as empowering in your authenticity, but often harder to say.

Therefore put on the whole armour of God, so that you may be able to withstand in the evil day, and having done all, to stand.

Ephesians 6:13

#50

Everything with Spiritual Wisdom

"You do not need to work to become spiritual. You are spiritual; you need only to remember that fact. Spirit is within you. God is within you."

Julia Cameron (1948-present)
American teacher, author, artist, poet, playwright, novelist, filmmaker, composer, and journalist.

"Hope is praying for rain, but faith is bringing an umbrella."

Unknown.

"Spirituality is not about being fixed; it is about God being present in the mess of our unfixedness."

Michael Yaconelli (1942-2003)
American writer and theologian, church leader, and satirist.

Some of the last words on the 'power potential wisdom' were about not being perfect, well the same is true in the last wisdom - in everything you do, have spiritual wisdom. Accept you'll never be spiritually perfect either. In this final wisdom I hope you have accepted that Ewald was a truly spiritual person and believed in a God, and in love for everyone and everything. To be spiritual you must believe in something, usually intangible, bigger and more powerful than you, that you never truly see or hear. In that belief you have to trust and be faithful. To get to the deeper levels of that takes wisdom, and it's not always easy when you've just lost your job, a family member just died, and you had a car accident on the way home. Being faithful in these instances is really tricky, and you need to be invested for the 'long-game.' Take some 'rough with the smooth'.

As Michael Yaconelli says *"...it is about God being present in the mess of our unfixedness."* Spiritual wisdom however is like a muscle, it needs work to make it better and stronger, you need to 'do stuff' to gain that wisdom. Reading your faith book, going to your faith building, and talking to the higher entity, (aka praying or meditation). Most importantly of all, you should live the values of your faith daily, hourly, every minute, and every second. Therein lies the crux and here endeth the lesson. Find your belief and faith, and embrace it, and live it daily. Standing in its power will also help.

For me as Christian, forever sinful and imperfect, reading my bible, going to church and praying is always time well spent. It always adds some wisdom I am lacking, and I am sure your faith can add the same to you. It doesn't have to be complicated. My shortest prayer in a day is usually *"Oh Lord help me"* then when I get stuck on something I usually ask myself *"What would Jesus do?"* Spiritual wisdom is there all the time, you just need to tap into it, and be prepared for the answer!

Life Hack #1

Meditation can help you reconnect you with your higher self and expand your spiritual awareness. Or pray and pray every day; and pray when you need something.

In the words of every Gen Z, - *"There is an App for that"* and there are plenty of apps for both meditation or praying and bible reading - commit to one if you're struggling with spirituality. Do something at the start and the end of every day, for spiritual wisdom.

Trust in the LORD with all your heart,
and do not lean on your own understanding.
In all your ways acknowledge Him, and He
will make straight your paths.

Proverbs 3:5-6

Acknowledgements

In helping me to stay true to Ewald's wisdom and in writing the book, I want to say a huge thank you to the following, all dear and valued colleagues in South Africa. Boetie and Jane Toerien, who were so much a part of Gail and Ewald Meggersee's journey and a part of the Body Stress Release community. Their kind words and dedication are always an inspiration to me; Brent Garvie, the guy who said *"Why don't you become a practitioner"* - thanks Brent I did, and you started my journey; Patti Blamire, who's wicked smile and wry sense of humour always keeps me real; Jeanette Gibbs, who until recently taught BSR at the Academy in Rondevlei and now devotes her *"spare time"*? to working for the BSR Foundation, she always keeps me sane with her straight talk and honesty. To Jean Holman, to whom I asked so many questions, never getting the answer I was looking for, but forever learning something new about everything in her head. Thanks also to Carolyn Shand for her inspiration to conceptualise the Meggersee Legacy Project, and her plan to capture the Meggersee's archival material, from her the idea to write this book was born and nurtured. To Martie-Louise Hunlun for checking various parts of the book, and ensuring coherence to the BSR brand, and the current Executive Committee (EXCO) members who also gave it a good once over!

Also, thanks to the BSR EXCO in South Africa for their permission to use the brand logo and in all their truly amazing voluntary work they do to support our 200+ practitioners in South Africa. It has been my honour and privilege to be their chairman up to the writing of this book. Thanks to Amanda Fourie,

Chairwoman of the BSR Foundation, and her amazing team, who supported this book. For each sale, a donation goes to funding their bursary scheme, which supports training practitioners less fortunate than others. They do amazing work in our previously disadvantaged and differently abled communities.

To the much wider 'kirk' of Body Stress Release practitioners worldwide, who are the most kind-hearted group of people I have had the honour to meet and work with for the last 10 years. For all BSR practitioners I hope this resonates with your memories of Ewald, and even if you didn't know him, I hope you find the clear and evident legacy of his wisdom and work in your most recent learning and understanding of the technique. All his wisdoms really are in the wonderful modality you practise.

To my book team, rather my 'Dream Team'; Wim Rheeder as ever grasped the design brief for a very different style to my previous history books, and came up with something lively for the format; Tony Sheffield for doing the editing and his laser focus for the English language, and for putting up with my many frustrating imperfections; Tony along with Martie-Louise Hunlun and Sandy Damant for their proof reading; and finally to Grant Walton from Castle Graphics, my brilliant printer for my third book with him in four years. Without all your work and help I would not be a self-publisher. Get ready for book 4, it is work-in-progress.

Love and Light

Simon

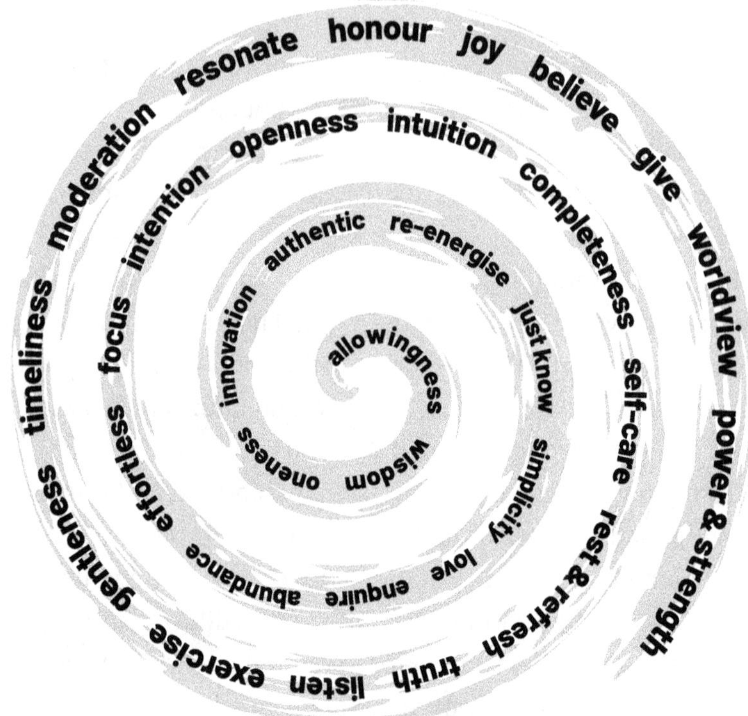

Final Word from Ewald

"My wish for everyone is that your journey to health may also be wonderous."

Ewald Meggersee
From *Self-Healing with Body Stress Release: Unlocking stored tension*
Gail Meggersee.

Bibliography

Angelou, Maya, *I Know Why the Caged Bird Sings*, Random House, 2009.

Baker, Tommy, *The 1% Rule: How to Fall in Love with the Process and Achieve Your Wildest Dreams*, Archangel Ink, 2018.

Bennett, Roy T, *The Light in the Heart: Inspirational Thoughts for Living Your Best Life*, Roy Bennett, 2020.

Bryson, Bill *The Body: A Guide for Occupants,* Penguin Random House UK, 2019.

Burchard, Brendon, *High Performance Habits*, Hay House Inc, 2022.

Byrne, Rhonda, *The Secret*, Atria Books, 2006.

Godin, Seth, *The Practice: Shipping Creative Work*, Penguin Business, 2020.

Coelho, Paulo, *The Alchemist*, HarperCollins Publishers, 2016.

Coelho, Paulo, *The Devil and Miss Prym*, HarperCollins Publishers, 2006.

Colgrove J, *The McKeown thesis: a historical controversy and its enduring influence*, American Journal of Public Health, May 2002.

Courtenay, Bryce, *The Power of One*, Random House, 1989.

Covey, Stephen R, *The 7 Habits of Highly Effective People*, Running Press, 2000.

Farooq, Raheel, *Why I Am a Muslim: And a Christian and a Jew,* independently published, 2020.

Gilbert, Elizabeth, *Eat Pray Love* , Penguin, 2006.

Goldberg, Natalie, *Writing down the Bones: Freeing the Writer Within*, Shambhala, 2005.

Goleman Daniel, *Emotional Intelligence: Why it can matter more than IQ*, Bantam Books, 1995.

Hawkins, David R, *Power vs. Force: The Hidden Determinants of Human Behaviour*, Hay House Inc, 1994.

Hay, Louise L, *Heal Your Body: The Mental Causes for Physical Illness and the Metaphysical Way to Overcome Them*, Hay House Inc, 1984.

Howes, Lewis, *The School of Greatness: A Real-World Guide to Living Bigger, Loving Deeper and Leaving a Legacy*, Rodale Books, 2017.

Karnazes, Dean, *Ultramarathon Man: Confessions of an All-Night Runner*, TarcherPerigee, 2006.

LePera, Dr Nicole, *How to Do the Work: Recognize Your Patterns, Heal from Your Past, and Create Your Self*, Collins, 2021.

Markides, Kyriacos C, *The Magus of Strovolos: The Extraordinary World of a Spiritual Healer*, Penguin Books, 1989.

Maxwell, John C, *Put Your Dreams to the Test, 10 Questions to Help You See it and Seize it*, Thomas & Nelson, 2009.

Maxwell, John C, *Good Leaders Ask Great Questions: Your Foundation for Successful Leadership*, Center Street, 2014.

McBride, Hillary L, *The Wisdom of Your Body: Finding Healing, Wholeness, and Connection through embodied Living*, Brazos Press, 2021.

Meggersee, Gail, *Self-Healing with Body Stress Release: Unlocking stored tension*, New Africa Books, 2007.

Mutwa, Credo, *Indaba, My Children: African Tribal History, Legends, Customs And Religious Beliefs*, Canongate Books Ltd, 1964.

Nin, Anaïs, *Delta of Venus*, Harcourt Brace Jovanovich, 1977.

Owen, Mark, *No Easy Day: The Autobiography of a Navy Seal: The Firsthand Account of the Mission That Killed Osama Bin Laden*, Dutton Books, 2012.

Peale, Norman Vincent, *The Power of Positive Thinking*, Cedar Books, 1990.

Peterson, Jordan B, *12 Rules for Life: An antidote to Chaos*, Penguin, 2018.

Ponder, Catherine, *The Dynamic Laws of Healing*, DeVorss Publications, 1996.

Robbins, Antony Jay, *Awaken The Giant Within: How to Take Immediate Control of Your Mental, Emotional, Physical and Financial Destiny!*, Simon & Schuster, 1991.

Robinson, Sir Ken, *The Element: How Finding Your Passion Changes Everything*, Penguin Books, 2010.

Roizen, Michael F, & Oz, Mehmet C, *You: The Owner's Manual: An Insider's Guide to the Body That Will Make You Healthier and Younger*, HarperCollins Publishers, 2005.

Roth, Emmanuel, James, *7 Strategies for Wealth and Health, Power Ideas from America's Foremost Business Philosopher*, Harmony, 1996.

Ruiz, Don Miguel, *The Four Agreements: A Practical Guide to Personal Freedom*, Amber-Allen Publishing, US 1997.

Sire, JW, *Naming the Elephant: Worldview as a Concept*, Intervarsity Press, 2004.

Stone, William Clement, *The Success System That Never Fails*, Martino Fine Books, 2017.

Tadevosyan, Arthur, *Croton: A Journey into the Afterlife*, Ozark Mountain Publishers, 2020.

Tamlyn, Rick, *Play Your Bigger Game: 9 Minutes to Learn, a Lifetime to Live*, Hay House, 2013.

Wilde, Oscar, *Oscar Wilde's Wit and Wisdom: A Book of Quotations,* Dover Publications Inc, 2000.

Winterson, Jeanette, *Oranges Are Not the Only Fruit*, Pandora Press, 1985.

Vaish, A., Grossmann, T., & Woodward, A. (2008). *Not all emotions are created equal: the negativity bias in social-emotional development*. Psychological bulletin, 134(3), 383–403. https://doi.org/10.1037/0033-2909.134.3.383

Van der Kolk, Bessel, *The Body Keeps the Score: Brain, Mind, and Body in the Healing of Trauma*, Penguin Books, 2015.

Wilde, Oscar, *The Picture of Dorian Gray*, Penguin Classics, 2003.

Other media

Meggersee, Ewald, Video BSR Academy, Presentation on Principles, 2010.

Holman, Jean, *BSR's DNA*, Inspiration Hour Presentation #26 to the BSR Community, 10 August 2024.

Holman, Jean, *The Mind Body Connection , BSR Workshop Notes,* 2022.

Robbins, Mel, Podcast Clips: How to Reprogram your Mind (RAS).

Websites

Above Down Inside Out philosophy.
https://www.drpolson.com/adio-above-down-inside-out/

Connected to self.
https://connectedtoself.com/healing-hack/

CreativeLive education platform.
www.chasejarvis.com/

Finding Your Resonant Frequency - Max Frenzel PhD.
https://medium.com/yudemon/finding-my-resonance-frequency-4e0eab189dfa

Healthiest Countries 2024 (Population Review).
https://worldpopulationreview.com/country-rankings/healthiest-countries

HeartMath Institute.
https://www.heartmath.org/

Hillary McBride website.
https://hillarylmcbride.com/books/

How Stuff Works - The Butterfly Effect
https://science.howstuffworks.com/math-concepts/butterfly-effect.htm

Institute for Health Metrics and Evaluation.
Global Burden of Disease Study (GBD) 2021.
https://www.healthdata.org/news-events/newsroom/news-releases/

NewScientist - The Duchenne Smile.
https://www.newscientist.com/definition/duchenne-smile/

Roads, Michael - website.
http://www.michaelroads.info/journey-into-the-secret-world-of-nature/

Rowse, Darren - aka ProBlogger.
https://problogger.com/about-darren/

Sir Ken Robinson website.
https://www.sirkenrobinson.com/

Statista Website - World Life Expectancy.
https://www.statista.com/statistics/1302736/global-life-expectancy-by-region-country-historical/

The Aesthetics of Joy.
https://aestheticsofjoy.com/why-the-secret-to-happiness-might-be-joy/

The Embassy of Good Science.
https://embassy.science/

World Health Index.
https://www.statista.com/statistics/1290168/health-index-of-countries-worldwide-by-health-index-score/

World Health Organization. Alcohol Statistics. Published May 9, 2022.
https://www.who.int/news-room/fact-sheets/detail/alcohol/

World Obesity Ranking.
https://data.worldobesity.org/rankings/

A selection of Ewald's Preferred Reading

Carlson, W Bernard, *Tesla: Inventor of the Electrical Age,* Princeton University Press, 2014.

Germinara, Gina, *Many Mansions: The Edgar Cayce Stroy on Reincarnation*, Signet, 1988.

Icke, David, *And the Truth Shall Set You Free: 21st Century Edition,* David Icke Books, 2004.

Klarer, Elizabeth, *Beyond the Light Barrier: The Autobiography of Elizabeth Klarer*, New Vision, 1980. 1980.

McClure, Rusty, *Coral Castle: The Mystery of Ed Leedskalnin and his American Stonehenge*, Ternary Publishing, 2009.

Roads, Michael J, *Talking with Nature and Journey into Nature,* HJ Kramer, 2003.

Roads, Michael J, *Journey Into Oneness and Into a Timeless Realm*, Six Degrees Publishing Group, 2015.

Schauberger, Viktor, *The Water Wizard: The Extraordinary Properties of Natural Water*, Gateway/Gill Books Publishing, 1999.

Tesla, Nikola, *Inventions, Researches and Writings of Nikola Tesla,* Kindle, 1970.

Willem, Alain, *Success DNA: how to clone greatness*, self-published, 2010.

Titles also available by Simon C Green

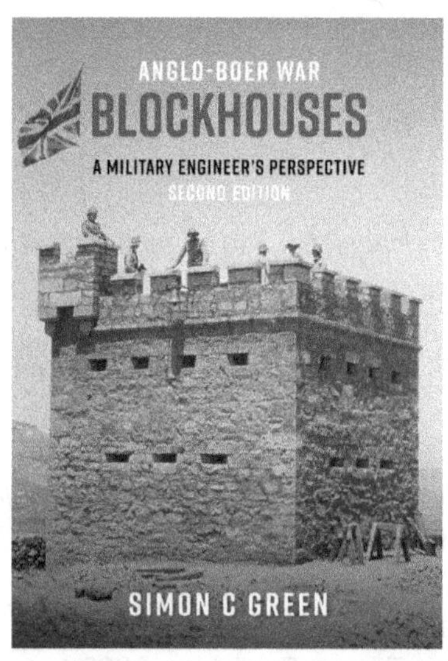

Anglo-Boer War Blockhouses:
A Military Engineer's Perspective (2nd Edition)
By Simon C Green

Anglo-Boer War Blockhouses: A Military Engineer's Perspective is a fresh analytical look at the how the construction of over 9 000 small fortifications during the Boer War sought to change its course. Apart from tracing the evolution of blockhouses elsewhere in the world, the book deals with the British Army's use of blockhouses prior to the war, to what conditions were like for the average "British Tommy" and his Imperial comrades fighting in these structures; it is a deep dive into the topic, previously not achieved.

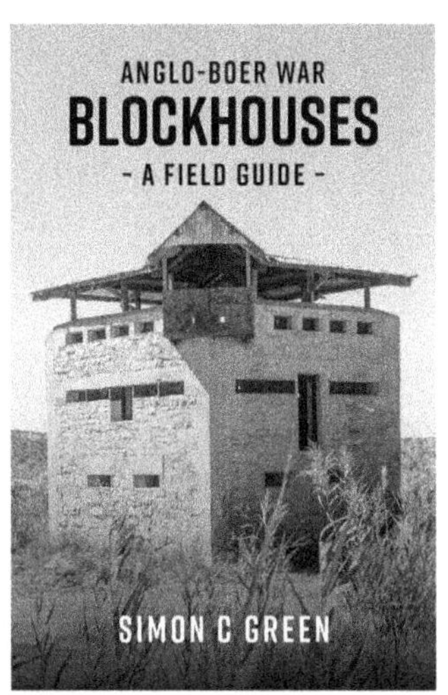

Anglo-Boer War Blockhouses: A Field Guide
By Simon C Green

The Field Guide, is a full colour companion to *Anglo-Boer War Blockhouses: A Military Engineer's Perspective*, and an extensive review of the blockhouses left standing in South Africa. A first-of-its-kind guide, it can be used for virtual visits to learn more about these military structures or better still to get 'boots on the ground'. Its aim is to put the blockhouse sites on the battlefield tour map and to encourage professional guides and amateurs alike to explore them or make them a stop-off on longer trips

To order books:
Visit www.blockhouses.co.za or Amazon for worldwide orders.

Or contact Simon for a signed copy or to speak at your event.
Email: simonbsr@gmail.com

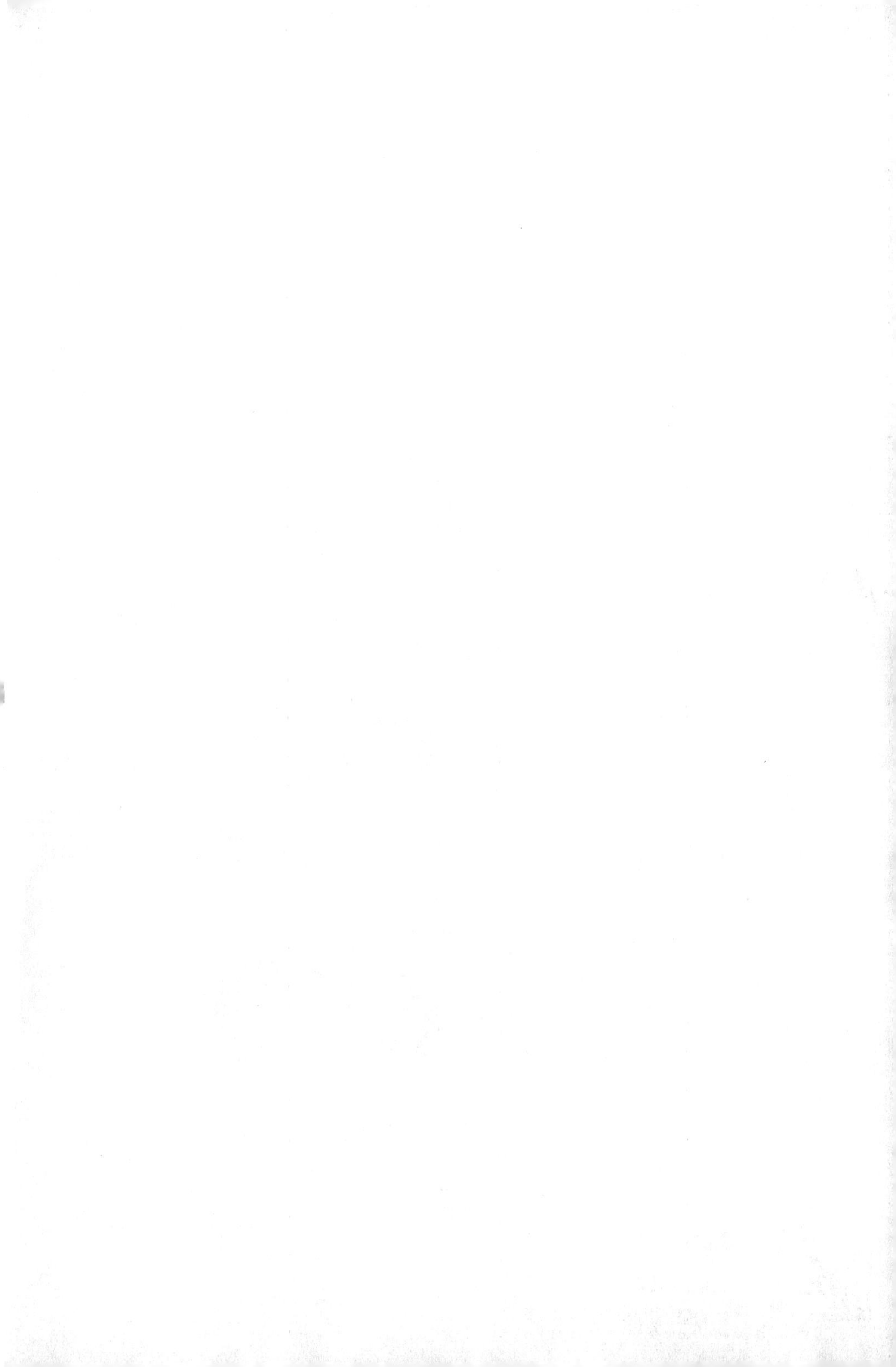

www.ingramcontent.com/pod-product-compliance
Lightning Source LLC
Chambersburg PA
CBHW070042040426
42333CB00041B/1955

* 9 7 8 1 0 3 7 0 3 2 6 2 2 *